READING AND UNDERSTANDING HEALTH RESEARCH

This concise guide equips readers with the essential skills required to analyze and critically appraise health research evidence, an integral element to evidence-based practice and professional development.

This book offers invaluable guidance by demystifying the structure and language of peer-reviewed research through different stages of reading—inspectional, analytical, and topical—to provide a structured approach to understanding and evaluating research design, methods, and findings. Through analytically reading each section of a research paper, readers can develop a critical appreciation of the evidence, helping them to identify both the strengths and limitations of any piece of research. This critical reading process is a crucial skill, fostering the ability to judiciously apply evidence to health practice, and encouraging a deep engagement with research to better inform health decisions.

Ideal reading for students across all health disciplines, whether undergraduate or postgraduate, it will also be a valuable resource for health professionals seeking to enhance their skills in evidence-based practice and continuing professional development. Instructors can also access a range of online resources to support classroom use.

Robert R. Weaver earned his doctoral degree in the Sociology of Health and Illness from the University of Connecticut, US. He currently teaches research methods in the Department of Health and Exercise Science (School of Nursing and Health Professions) at Rowan University, US.

Qian Jia earned her doctoral degree in Nutrition from Texas A&M University, US, and is a registered dietitian. She currently teaches Interprofessional Healthcare Research and Graduate Nutrition Capstone courses in the College of Nursing and Health Professions at Immaculata University, US.

READING AND UNDERSTANDING HEALTH RESEARCH

A Critical Approach

Robert R. Weaver and Qian Jia

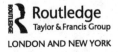

Routledge
Taylor & Francis Group

LONDON AND NEW YORK

Designed cover image: Getty Images

First published 2025
by Routledge
4 Park Square, Milton Park, Abingdon, Oxon, OX14 4RN

and by Routledge
605 Third Avenue, New York, NY 10158

Routledge is an imprint of the Taylor & Francis Group, an informa business

© 2025 Robert R. Weaver and Qian Jia

British Library Cataloguing-in-Publication Data
A catalogue record for this book is available from the British Library

ISBN: 978-1-032-97831-4 (hbk)
ISBN: 978-1-032-23009-2 (pbk)
ISBN: 978-1-003-59566-3 (ebk)

DOI: 10.4324/9781003595663

Typeset in Sabon
by codeMantra

Access the Support Material: www.routledge.com/9781032230092

CONTENTS

FIGURES

TABLES

BOXES

ACKNOWLEDGMENTS

Robert: I wish to express my gratitude for the opportunity to engage with so many students and colleagues in discussions about the roles science can play for improving human health. Special thanks go to Ayush, Otto, Shilpa, Rob, and Nicole. I am sincerely grateful to colleagues at Rowan University's Department of Health and Exercise Science for providing such a stimulating and thoroughly pleasant place to work. Research students have provided important feedback on different versions of this manuscript. Particular thanks go to Leah Crilly who carefully read and helped edit the final version. I owe much to Qian, an outstanding health scientist from whom I have learned a great deal, and who has proven to be an even better colleague and collaborator. Above all, I am grateful for my partner in life and love, Nawal, for her patience and support during the many hours I spent on this project. My daughter, Soraya, not only contributed creatively to various figures in this document but has also brought immeasurable joy and fulfillment to my life.

Qian: I am profoundly grateful to all my undergraduate and graduate students, whose inspiration has fueled this project, and to my colleagues at Immaculata University's College of Nursing and Health Professions for fostering a warm and supportive academic environment. I would also like to express my sincere appreciation to my graduate advisors at Texas A&M University, Dr. Robert Chapkin and Dr. David McMurray, for guiding my understanding of scientific methodology during my graduate studies. Lastly, I extend my heartfelt gratitude to my three wonderful children, Cody (14), Carlo (12), and Camille (4), for their cooperation throughout this project, and to my life partner, Jacky, for his unwavering love and encouragement in all my endeavors.

Initialisms and acronyms

CDC – Centers for Disease Control
CI – confidence interval
EBP – Evidence-Based Practice
MMWR – Morbidity and Mortality Weekly Report
NHANES – National Health And Nutrition Examination Survey
ORs, RRs, and HRs – Odds ratio, Risk Ratio, and Hazard Ratios.
RCT – Randomized Controlled Trial

PREFACE

In an increasingly crowded and changing information landscape, the capacity to critically read and understand health science research becomes indispensable for both emerging and established health professionals. This manuscript, *Reading and Understanding Health Research: A Critical Approach*, addresses the need for students and health professionals to take an active, analytical approach to effectively and critically consuming research evidence to inform evidence-based practice and to promote professional growth.

As a health science student transitioning into the health professions, you may already recognize that learning to read critically is an ongoing process throughout your academic and professional careers. This ongoing learning is crucial not only for understanding and applying the most current and effective scientific evidence to your practice decisions but also for your long-term professional development. It involves mastering better ways to critically evaluate and utilize research evidence before advising on or making health-related decisions. Indeed, as the volume and pace of information exchange accelerates, the ability to critically scrutinize health science research becomes more and more important.

The challenges and complexities of reading health research require the ongoing development and refinement of critical reading skills. Like most difficult tasks, reading research articles is hardest for the beginner, but that is also where the learning curve is steepest and the greatest gains are achieved. We recommend that health professionals engage in the process of critically reading and consuming research evidence "early and often". Cultivating the habit of inspecting articles to identify those that do and do not align with one's reading aim, critically analyzing only the most relevant ones, and summarizing and synthesizing the findings from multiple studies broaden and deepen the professional's understanding of the topic of interest. It is the habit of critically reading and analyzing health science research that underlies evidence-based practice and growth as a health professional.

We hope that this book serves as a valuable resource for health science students and health professionals, equipping them with the approach and the skills necessary to critically engage with scientific research, make evidence-based decisions, and grow as professionals. By fostering critical reading, this book aims to contribute to the culture of evidence-based practice that is responsive to the complexities of modern healthcare.

Robert R. Weaver & Qian Jia
September, 2024

1

INTRODUCTION

Reading health science

Professional growth and evidence-based practice (EBP)

Health professionals are expected to apply the best available scientific evidence in serving clients or patients. Clients surely expect that and so do fellow professionals. The best available evidence comes from peer-reviewed scientific studies. These studies inform professional guidelines for engaging in practice based on scientific evidence.

Yet even the best evidence does not apply equally to all patients or clients. Thus, understanding the limits of the evidence and the particulars of each unique individual – e.g., their values, preferences, and health capabilities – is essential for assessing how general evidence might apply to an individual case. As shown in Figure 1.1, EBP involves (1) understanding relevant evidence, (2) understanding the unique qualities of individual cases, and (3) drawing on professional experience and judgment to reconcile the two.

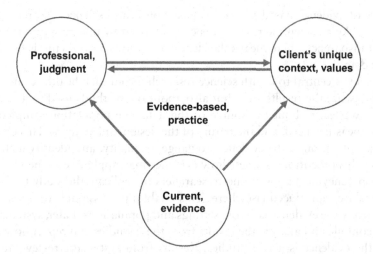

FIGURE 1.1   Evidence-based practice (EBP) – evidence, professional judgment, and the client's uniqueness.

DOI: 10.4324/9781003595663-1

For example, when a nurse in a hospital is tasked with preventing pressure ulcers in bedridden patients, the nurse might refer to the guideline developed by the National Pressure Ulcer Advisory Panel for guidance on risk assessment and skin assessment. The nurse may also determine the most effective intervention by conducting a literature review to gather evidence on various preventive measures. Based on this evidence from the guideline and literature review, the hospital may implement a protocol requiring that nurses reposition bedridden patients every 2 hours. However, the patient may refuse to follow this protocol during night to maintain sleep. The nurse and the healthcare team will need to engage in open communication with the patient to understand the reason for refusal and to address any concerns or barriers to decision making. The healthcare team may need to educate the patient regarding the short-term and long-term treatment goals and engage the patient in shared decision-making by discussing alternative options or compromises that align with both the patient's preferences and the hospital's protocol.

Sourcing and critically assessing evidence from research literature is an invaluable skill that healthcare professionals will cultivate to foster a practice that is evidence-based. This book aims to equip readers with a structured framework for understanding, analyzing, and confidently utilizing the latest evidence in their clinical practice.

Following this introduction, this book describes the process of searching for and inspecting peer-reviewed research articles (Part 1) and analytically reading primary research articles (Part 2) and systematic reviews (Part 3). Part 4 describes the process of "topical" reading, where research evidence on a topic is characterized, interpreted, and synthesized.

In addition to describing findings as presented in research articles, the critical reader analyzes these findings with respect to the methods used to produce them, identifies biases they might contain, and the limitations of their applications. Critically reading health research is inextricably tied to any practice that is evidence-based.

Health science methods and evidence

The evidence of evidence-based practice is based on health science research. Health science research, like all scientific research, is characterized by openness and transparency. The term "transparency" here means the clear description of the methods used to collect and analyze data.

Transparency is central to health science research. From each health science study, we learn not only what the results were but also about the methods used to generate them. For instance, we learn about the source of the data, the population sampled, the reliability of the measures used, and the nature of the design and analysis. This enables us to refine our interpretation of the evidence, to gauge its quality, and identify its limitations. In turn, this helps practitioners assess how evidence may apply in each new situation.

This transparency also allows other researchers to replicate the study to determine if similar results are reproduced elsewhere. This enables professionals to assess how consistent and strong the evidence is across settings and populations. Later, systematic review studies will compile and analyze the results from these studies and report how consistent and strong the evidence is across studies. Results from systematic review studies often come to inform existing professional practice guidelines (Chapter 13).

Reading health science research

Peer-reviewed articles

To date, peer-reviewed articles serve as the major vehicle for health scientists to communicate research findings from health science studies. A main feature of peer-reviewed articles is their transparency in reporting study methods and findings. This transparency enables others to critically analyze the findings in terms of their validity and applicability.

Critical analysis requires a cautious approach in assessing their validity and determining where they might apply. Keeping a skeptical orientation rather than accepting what you read at face value is challenging, especially for early professionals. Articles are mainly written by and for experts in the field already versed in the vocabulary of the subject matter and the language of methods (see Box 1.1). They are not written for the typical undergraduate or even graduate student. At the same time, it offers an opportunity for early professionals to expand their vocabulary, learn the language of health science, and gain a clearer grasp of the nature and quality of evidence on a health topic.

BOX 1.1 THE CURSE OF KNOWLEDGE

The curse of knowledge is the assumption authors make about the knowledge and background of an audience of readers. The curse often appears when young health practitioners encounter health research articles that have been authored by experts to an audience of other experts. Critically analyzing research articles becomes a challenge for young health professionals with little training and experience. Little is gained, however, by reading material you already know, while learning the language and issues from experts in your area of interest advances professional growth: "an article that is over your head is one that can teach you something" [1].

Basic concepts and terms

There is no side-stepping the fact that reading peer-reviewed articles requires learning the concepts and vocabulary of their chosen field along with the methods used to generate knowledge in that field. The learning curve is hardest for the beginner but also where the curve is steepest.

Terms that are unfamiliar usually reflect the level of training and your exposure to them, not their complexity or an ability to grasp their meaning. Many unfamiliar terms can be understood from the context in which they are found, by searching online for descriptions, or simply from continued exposure to them. Expanding one's vocabulary occurs naturally as one actively consumes health research and interacts with professional colleagues. An expanding vocabulary is one sign of professional growth.

Apart from learning basic terms about the topic, early professionals will see how these terms fit within the larger narrative of the research article. The structure of this narrative is similar across fields and subfields of health research (see Chapter 4). Articles begin with a rationale, describe the methods used to collect and analyze data, and present findings and conclusions.

BOX 1.2 TWO SETS OF TERMS

Research articles contain at least two distinct sets of terms. One set pertains to the health issue one wishes to explore – e.g., a health outcome such as diabetes, injury, or mental health. To learn and understand the evidence that pertains to the specific health issue is primarily what we read for. A second set of terms pertains to the research methods used to generate evidence surrounding the health issues – e.g., the research design, sampling strategies, variable measures, analytic strategies. These terms cut across all substantive areas in health science. Understanding these terms is crucial for critically assessing the findings from research articles. Appendix A identifies some elementary terms that pertain to these research methods.

Reading stages and process

Reading peer-reviewed research articles is challenging, especially for younger, less experienced professionals (see Box 1.2). The reading process divides into four phases: (1) elementary reading, (2) inspectional reading, (3) analytical reading, and (4) topical reading [1]:

1 **Elementary reading.** Elementary reading pertains to learning basic terms and language, in this case of research methods and of subject matter related to health and illness. Elementary reading is an ongoing process that occurs as one grows as a person and professional (see Appendix A for a list of key research terms).
2 **Inspectional reading.** Obviously, the aims of the article should align as much as possible with your aim or purpose of reading. This alignment can be assessed quickly by inspecting the article's title and abstract. Inspectional reading involves discerning the relevance of the research study to the reading aim based on a careful assessment of the study's title and abstract (see Chapters 3 and 4).
3 **Analytical reading.** Analytic reading involves critically reading key elements of methods the study used to collect and analyze data. The quality and utility of a study's findings are determined by the nature and quality of the methods used to generate them. Analytical reading is critical for effective, evidence-based decision making and practice (see Parts 2 and 3).
4 **Topical reading.** Topical reading is the highest stage of reading, where the evidence from several studies is interpreted, synthesized, and applied to health decisions and actions that are evidence based (see Part 4).

These four levels of reading also reflect the process involved when health professionals inquire and wish to learn more about a topic or health problem

1 define the aim of reading – learn elementary terms of research to assist in searching for relevant studies;

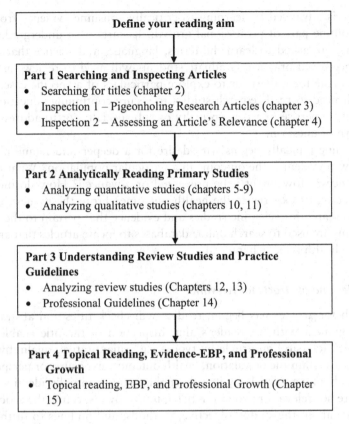

FIGURE 1.2   The process of reading – inspectional, analytical, and topical, and the chapter sequence.

2 critically inspect titles and abstracts of records returned to determine studies you wish to analyze (inspectional reading);

3 critically analyze relevant studies to assess the findings and limitations of each (analytical reading);

4 summarize, interpret, and synthesize the evidence from multiple studies on the topic (topical reading).

The flowchart shown in Figure 1.2 captures this process and informs the organization of this book.

Defining the topic of the inquiry and searching for relevant studies

Drawing on and applying the best available evidence to practice decisions in the service of clients will motivate reading science research. However, critically reading and consuming research evidence underlies the ongoing process of professional development. Undergraduate and graduate training, internships, apprenticeships, practical experience, continuous education, and engagement with current research all enhance one's ability to interact with professional colleagues and inform a practice that is evidence based.

This ability is advanced by learning to critically consume evidence from health research as a routine part of professional growth. It starts with undergraduate training, where students are asked to learn the terms, language, and science that drive professional, evidence-based practice. Graduate students will need to review the literature to provide a rationale for a thesis or to explore particulars of a specific case. Health professionals will need to read research studies to secure continuing education credits, or to develop new expertise in a new specialty or sub-specialty, or to address a particular client's concern or question.

Critical reading typically begins with desire for a deeper understanding of a health outcome. How prevalent is the outcome in a particular population? What are its causes and consequences? How might it be prevented or advanced? How do individuals understand, perceive, or experience the health outcome? From these questions come key words used to search for scientific studies and evidence that pertain to the health topic. These key terms are used to search online databases to locate articles that are potentially relevant to the health issue (Chapter 2).

Inspecting titles and abstracts for relevance

Once a search for articles has begun, readers will check titles and abstracts to determine their alignment with the reader's aim. Inspection of the title enables the reader to "pigeonhole" (classify) an article by type – e.g., quantitative, qualitative, or review study – and to ascertain the population, health outcome, exposure, or perspectives being studied. Pigeonholing an article by its title enables you to initially identify and exclude articles that are not relevant to your aim (Chapter 3). By inspecting the article's abstract, you learn more about the study's objective, methods, and findings to further assess the study's relevance to your reading aim (Chapter 4). Taking time to inspect the abstract helps you to exclude articles from the inquiry, leaving only those considered relevant to your aim to a thorough, critical analysis.

The more one understands research methods, the more effective, focused, and refined the search will become. The more practice one has in inspecting research articles, the more focused the search process will become.

Analyzing research studies for quality

Going beyond the title and abstract, analytic reading involves critically examining the body of an article, especially the methods and results. Understanding the nature and quality of the methods used to generate findings enhances your critical understanding of the findings and their application to practice decisions.

Articles begin with a rationale for conducting the study (Chapter 4). This involves describing the need for the research and the objectives of the current study. Here again the readers can assess the relevance of the study for their particular purpose.

The description of methods used to collect and analyze data is the chief focus of analytically reading an article. To assess the quality of findings, one needs to understand the methods used to collect and analyze data. Chapters 5–11 describe designs used to critically analyze primary studies – observational, experimental, and qualitative.

Health professionals increasingly rely on evidence from review studies as well – i.e., studies that compare, contrast, and synthesize results from several primary studies (Chapter 12). Review studies have also become more transparent in describing the selection and assessment of studies for review, the extraction of findings, and the analysis and synthesis of these findings. Health professionals will rely on evidence from systematic reviews and practice to inform their practice (Chapters 12 and 13).

Health professionals will also rely on practice guidelines to shape their practice (Chapter 14). Practice guidelines are developed by professional associations to guide professional practice in high-priority areas in public health and healthcare. They are based on an expert review of current evidence on important topics to help guide the decisions and actions of professionals and the public.

Topical reading – interpreting results from several studies

Health professionals do not necessarily change their practices based on results of a single primary or review study. Additionally, there might not be a practice guideline to help address the specifics of the health topic of concern. Rather, health professionals need to critically review and interpret results from several studies and decide how evidence applies to practice decisions or actions. The critical review of research evidence involves the highest stage of reading – "topical" reading (Chapter 15).

Topical reading compares, summarizes, and synthesizes findings from several studies – e.g., "5 articles found this, 7 articles found that, and 3 articles found something else". However, topical reading encompasses more. Besides comparing studies and describing the results, topical reading combines and interprets what the evidence means and how it may apply in everyday practice.

Topical reading continues throughout one's career and, with time and practice, professionals learn to assess evidence and its utility with growing discernment and effectiveness. This is central to professional growth, which, in turn, forms the foundation for evidence-based practice.

Recap

Chapter 1 has introduced the relationship between professional growth and evidence-based practice (EBP), and highlights the role critically reading health research plays in cultivating both. Specifically, it argued that peer-reviewed health science research offers the most valid, reliable, and up-to-date source of health-related scientific evidence and is, therefore, central for EBP. The chapter then described key stages of reading – inspectional, analytical, and topical reading – each stage building on the one before.

These stages of reading help to structure the entire book. Understanding and practicing inspectional, analytical, and topical reading provides a foundation for continuous learning, evidence-based practice, and professional growth.

Reference

1. Adler MJ, van Doren C. *How to read a book: The classic guide to intelligent reading*. New York: Simon and Schuster; 1972.

PART 1

Searching and inspecting articles

Part 1 of this book describes the inspectional phase of reading a peer-reviewed research article. It describes how readers can locate research articles and efficiently determine their relevance to the professional's larger reading aim. To determine the relevance of an article, readers first identify their aim or purpose of reading, often broadly expressed as a health topic.

Once the general reading aim has been identified Chapter 2 introduces the basic ingredients of effective searches for health research articles. It emphasizes the importance of breaking down a health topic into three key components: the health outcome, the population affected, and the exposure or intervention. These components form the basis of search terms that can be used to navigate databases like PubMed effectively. The Chapter guides the reader on how to use search filters and Boolean operators to refine search results, ensuring that only the most relevant articles are identified.

Chapter 3 describes the inspectional stage of reading where titles of peer-reviewed research articles are first "inspected" for their relevance to the purpose of reading aim. The Chapter outlines key distinctions that can be made to pigeonhole the health text by its type – e.g., is it peer-reviewed? Is it a primary or review study? Is a quantitative or qualitative approach taken? Determining an article's relevance also requires identifying its topic. By parsing and extracting information from the title, readers can also learn the outlines of the study's topic – the health outcome, exposure, population, or experience being explored. The process of parsing titles helps readers to exclude the myriad health-related texts that are irrelevant to their topic of concern.

Chapter 4 extends the discussion of inspectional reading to include an examination of the study's abstract. The abstract provides an overview of the entire study, its aim, methods, key findings, and major implications. The abstract is typically sufficient to give readers the essential content of the study and help them decide whether the study deserves the more in-depth, analytical reading required to assess how the evidence provided may apply to practice.

DOI: 10.4324/9781003595663-2

By mastering these foundational skills, health professionals can better navigate the vast and complex landscape of health research to identify relevant articles that align with their reading purpose.

2

FINDING RELEVANT ARTICLES

Searching for articles to inspect – health outcomes, populations, and exposures

Health-related studies and information reach us without the need for active searching. Some may sound interesting, but most are marginally relevant to anything we really need to know about a specific health issue. This passive consumption of "findings" from random studies, particularly without critically analyzing the methods used to generate them, is potentially harmful to practice or, at best, a waste of time.

The passive consumption of research as it presents itself sits in contrast to an active and deliberate approach, where the health topic or issue one wishes to learn about is first defined, and research evidence surrounding the issue is critically examined and interpreted. There are countless questions or health issues that might be of concern, prompted by personal or professional circumstances. Some questions may seek descriptive information about some attribute of a population: "what is the incidence and prevalence of type-2 diabetes among Asian Americans?". These questions aim to describe characteristics of a group or population.

Other questions or issues may seek evidence about the association between exposures and outcomes. For instance, athletic trainers might ask: "what are the risk factors associated with ACL injury among college athletes?". A dietitian might ask: "what is the effect of a diet intervention on heart health among adults 50 years old and older?" These questions can break down into three key search terms: outcomes (e.g., type-2 diabetes, ACL injury, and heart health), exposures (e.g., risk factors and diet intervention), and populations (e.g., Asian Americans, college athletes, and adults over 50).

More generally, defining the health issue or topic of concern may be broken down into three major components

1 The health outcome – the physical or mental health condition that should be fostered, mitigated, or better understood;

DOI: 10.4324/9781003595663-3

2 Specific population or group – the population or group that experiences the outcome, or where the outcome is or is not prevalent;

3 An exposure – a natural exposure that is associated with the outcome (e.g., a risk factor) or a treatment intervention designed to rehabilitate, mitigate, or foster the health outcome.

The reader's task is to identify meaningful keywords associated with the question or topic to create an online search that delivers articles worth inspecting and critically analyzing.

BOX 2.1 RESEARCH DESIGN AS A KEY TERM

Different research designs produce varying findings on the same health topic. For instance, a cross-sectional study of ACL injury would provide information about the prevalence of the injury whereas a randomized control trial (RCT) would test the effectiveness of a treatment program designed to repair the ACL. Findings from a qualitative design might describe the experiences and challenges of the ACL injury recovery process. Parts 2 and 3 of this text are structured around research designs and the kind of evidence each design yields. As you refine your reading aim and become more practiced in your queries you will add a research design to the string of key terms used to locate relevant studies.

Online searches (PubMed)

The health issue or topic that motivates an inquiry must be translated into search terms or keywords that can be used to locate abstracts and articles available in online databases. PubMed is an online database that is widely used by health scientists and practitioners.

For instance, you may wish to use PubMed to locate articles about risk factors associated with ACL injury among women's basketball players. Searches using ACL injury (health outcome) and basketball (exposure), among college women (population) (Table 2.1).

Using only one keyword to capture the health outcome – ACL injury – returned 21,297 titles. Sorting through all these titles to identify the few that might be relevant would be virtually impossible. When paired with an exposure – college basketball – the number diminished markedly to 58. When the search is further restricted by population – "women" – the number of titles returned decreased to 20. Finally, filtering these results by publication date – e.g., to studies published within the last 5 years – the number of returns further declines to four titles.

TABLE 2.1 PubMed search history with health outcome, exposure, and population

Search history	Title returned
#1 – ACLinjury	21,297
#2 – (#1) and (college basketball)	58
#3 – (#2) and (women)	20
#4 – (#3) and (in the last 5 years	4

The health outcome, exposure, and target population are basic terms used to define a health issue and search. Subsequent chapters will discuss how different research designs yield different types of evidence. Thus, a search may be further refined to target the quality of evidence you might be seeking (see Box 2.1).

Search filters and online databases

Search filters

Search tools include filters that are used to narrow the search and reduce the number of irrelevant titles returned. The search may be limited to include only those articles where keywords appear in the title or abstract. They may also be limited to studies published within the last 1, 5, or 10 years or within a specific window of time. In addition, the search may be restricted by age, gender, geographic region, or language.

Search filters, along with the careful selection and arrangement of keywords (Box 2.2), provide a range of options to enable the identification of titles that promise to address your research interest (see the PubMed User Guide). Once titles are located, the process of carefully inspecting the titles and abstracts for relevance begins (Chapters 3 and 4).

BOX 2.2   BOOLEAN OPERATORS – "AND", "OR" OR "NOT"

Searches can be expanded or limited by connecting keywords by Boolean operators such as "AND" or "OR". "AND" means that both keywords must be included for the title to be retrieved. "OR" means that either keyword may be present for the title to be retrieved. A search for articles that included ACL injury "AND" ankle injury retrieved 261 results. A search for articles that included ACL injury "OR" ankle injury retrieved 14,335 results. The operator "NOT" is also frequently used to explicitly exclude retrieval terms from the search. It can serve as another filter in the search. For instance, you may wish to exclude review studies from the search to retrieve only primary research studies.

Online databases

There are several online databases to draw from in searching for studies relevant to your topic. The databases may vary in terms of the journals and topics they are likely to include, though there is overlap among them. Online databases include journals suitable to some professionals rather than others. For instance, nurses and dietitians may search PubMed and CINAHL, whereas physical and occupational therapists will mainly use PubMed and PEDro.

Here are four major sources of online databases

1   *Academic libraries* provide robust access to several searchable databases that serve different areas of interest. To serve the health professions (e.g., public health, nursing, medicine, kinesiology, sports, physical and occupational therapy), commonly used databases include Public Health Database, PubMed, CINAHL, SPORTDiscus, Cochrane

Reviews, ProQuest, PsychInfo, and OVID. The downside is that practicing professionals who are not affiliated with a university may not have access to them.

2 *Professional associations* often provide access to journals, practice guidelines, and other resources specific to the profession. Associations may restrict access to just its dues-paying members. Apart from online databases, individual health professionals may also stay current by subscribing to selected journals in their specialty area.

3 *PubMed (and PMC)* provides access to abstracts or the full text of research articles for anyone connected to the internet. It is widely known and used and offers an open-access database funded by the US's National Institutes of Health/National Library of Medicine. It enables access to article titles and abstracts, and the full-text for those published in open-access journals. PubMed Central (PMC) is another NLM-sponsored database that includes full-text articles.

4 The *Google Scholar* database provides links to the title and abstract of academic articles available, and to full-text articles from open-access journals. It can be convenient for very quick searches but is less so for developing more advanced searches often required to zero-in on the most relevant articles. Further, the number of records returned is often too many to wade through. The same search that yielded 28 hits using the CINAHL database, yielded 6,500 using Google Scholar.

Differences in the number of titles returned using the same basic keyword search in all four databases are shown in Table 2.2.

The table shows the value of using online databases designed to target health issues rather than using Google Scholar. Anyone interested in risk factors for ACL injury among female college basketball players are looking at 266 titles on the topic, a fraction of which will be relevant to the reader. Common online health databases yielded a manageable number of potentially relevant articles to "pigeonhole" (Chapter 3).

Online databases have their own user interfaces, but once you learn the essential logic and options available, you will soon learn to navigate them. As suggested above, Google Scholar provides a very blunt instrument for locating health science articles, often returning an unmanageable number of titles. Other databases may not be available to anyone not connected to a health research institution.

PubMed provides ready access to over 5,000 journals and tens of millions of abstracts and citations. Unlike many specialized databases, it does not require affiliation with a large library or research institution. PubMed also provides links to millions of full-text articles through PubMed Central (PMC), a free full-text archive of life and health science literature.

TABLE 2.2 Keyword search and titles returned using different online databases

Search string	# Results returned			
	Google Scholar	SPORTDiscus	CINAHL	PubMed
#1 = ACL injury	45.9 K	3.5 K	6.8 K	21.3 K
#2 = #1 AND college basketball	365	17	7	58
#3 = #2 AND women	266	8	3	20

With a changing information landscape due to the deployment of artificial intelligence (AI) tools, new ways of searching and finding information to inform decisions will likely emerge (Box 2.3). Yet at their core, topics of human health and illness will still involve an understanding of how to address a given health problem, and this involves understanding their prevalence, causes, risks, and the various human effects certain actions might likely have. Understanding what it is you are looking for and why is more fundamental than the tools you use for finding it.

BOX 2.3   ON AI USE IN HEALTH PRACTICE

It is early days, but artificial intelligence (AI) tools may soon serve the health professional as another important tool to inform decisions. Unlike peer-reviewed studies, however, AI tools lack transparency so we cannot know where their responses come from – e.g., what training data did they learn from, what algorithms were used to analyze the data and generate their human-like responses. In short, we cannot know what biases underlie their responses. Instead, what AI tools offer is akin to a supercharged "narrative review" (Chapter 12). Although narrative reviews are often useful, they do not replace peer-reviewed studies as the "gold standard" for health science evidence.

Recap

This Chapter outlined the central components of the online search process designed for health professionals seeking high-quality evidence to inform health decisions. It suggested the importance of breaking down a health topic into its essential elements for guiding a search – the health outcome, the population or group affected, and the exposure or intervention.

The chapter described the use of search keywords and filters (e.g., publication year, population age and gender, research design) to narrow search results to studies that are more relevant to the topic. As students and health professionals deepen their understanding of research terms and methods, their searches will become even more targeted, including research designs to enhance the relevance of the studies returned from the search. The strategic use of search terms and filters effectively narrows the focus of the search, excluding studies of limited relevance from consideration. An effective search strategy serves as the first step toward efficiently locating studies and evidence designed to inform health decisions and actions.

3

INSPECTION 1

Pigeonholing an article by its title

Overview – inspecting health-related texts

The universe of health-related texts includes any written material that makes some claim about the prevalence, incidence, causes, consequences, experiences, or remedies related to some health issue. This includes online posts, media messages, news reports, commentaries, books, gray literature, advertisements as well as peer-reviewed research articles. Given their diverse origins and purposes, the quality and accuracy of health texts varies greatly. They can misinform as well as inform the consumer.

A critical distinction exists between peer-reviewed and non-peer-reviewed research. Peer-reviewed research undergoes rigorous review by expert peers before being published. This peer-review process serves as a quality control mechanism, where independent scholars critically assess study's methodology, data analysis, and conclusions. The process ensures that the research meets specific standards of validity, reliability, and academic integrity. As a result, peer-reviewed articles are widely regarded as the most credible and trustworthy source of information, forming the foundation of evidence-based practice decisions and actions.

Peer-reviewed research also requires transparency – a clear, explicit description of the research findings and the methods used to generate them. This openness is necessary for peer reviewers to assess the quality of the research. Results are not taken at face value. Instead, the quality of the results can be assessed based on the quality of the methods used to produce them.

Transparency also allows other researchers to replicate and verify results. Thus, transparency fosters accountability in research, the accumulation of evidence on the topic, and the expansion of health-related knowledge and understanding.

In contrast, other health-related texts are less transparent and will make claims that cannot be readily verified. They have not survived a rigorous peer-review process. Any health-related claims and the findings they are based upon must be taken at face value. Typically, online posts, media messages, and other health-related texts present

DOI: 10.4324/9781003595663-4 ·

results, conclusions, or opinions without describing how or where they came from. While non-peer-reviewed sources can offer valuable insights and timely information (see Box 3.1), they often lack the rigorous validation that characterizes peer-reviewed studies. Consequently, the reliability and accuracy of non-peer-reviewed research can vary widely, and these sources may sometimes disseminate misinformation or unfounded claims.

In sum, having survived a rigorous review process, peer-reviewed research remains the gold standard for credible and reliable health information. Hence, this book focuses on a subset of health-related texts – peer-reviewed articles that provide evidence designed to inform health practice that is evidence-based.

BOX 3.1   NON-PEER-REVIEWED HEALTH TEXTS

Although many health texts are intentionally or unintentionally misleading or designed to promote commercial interests, some may inform or inspire peer-reviewed research. Anecdotal reports can draw attention to emergent health problems and provide a context for formulating ideas or testing hypotheses. Reports from industry, think tanks, or from governmental agencies can steer research in specific directions. Two monumental reports – *To Err is Human* and *Crossing the Quality Chasm* [1, 2] – are said to have inspired the patient safety movement. While we draw a sharp distinction between peer-reviewed and non-peer-reviewed research, the boundary between the two remains porous.

Inspecting article titles

Inspectional reading attempts to gain an overview of the study, where it fits amid other health-related studies. Inspectional reading enables the reader to rapidly exclude irrelevant studies from consideration and bring the focus to the more relevant ones. Although it takes little time, inspectional reading saves a lot of time and energy considering studies that are of marginal relevance to the reader's aim.

For instance, in a rapidly evolving information landscape, the recency of research findings becomes critical. By simply noting the year of publication helps the reader exclude studies likely to be outdated or superseded by more current research. Excluding older research studies (which often is accomplished beforehand with a search filter), turns the focus to the title of the study. Article titles are often long, include subtitles, and are densely packed. They are dense because they contain valuable information about the study. Carefully reading titles enables readers to discover:

1 what *type* of study is contained in the article, and
2 what *topic-related* information the study examined.

Each is discussed in turn.

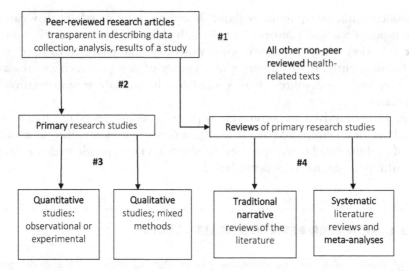

FIGURE 3.1   Four key distinctions used to pigeonhole research articles by type of study being described.

Pigeonholing article titles by *type*

Once an article's recency has been established, inspectional reading involves parsing the title of the study to identify key terms that allow the study to be placed in a larger context of all health-related texts. Figure 3.1 provides a flowchart of the initial distinctions active readers make to pigeonhole health texts during the inspection phase of reading.

The figure identifies several fundamental distinctions that allow readers to compartmentalize health research studies.

1 Distinction #1 – between peer-reviewed research articles and all other health-related texts that have not been peer reviewed
2 Distinction #2 – peer-reviewed articles that describe a primary study and those that describe a review study
3 Distinction #3 – primary studies that take a quantitative approach and those that take a qualitative approach
4 Distinction #4 – review studies that describe a traditional narrative review and those that describe a systematic review.

Pigeonholing an article by its title enables the readers to promptly distinguish between studies that align with their reading aim and those that do not. This differentiation becomes crucial amid the diverse array of health texts available.

Distinction 1: Peer-reviewed research or not

Those actively seeking up-to-date health information and evidence that is valid and reliable will look to identify peer-reviewed research articles from the diverse array of health-related texts one may encounter. As described earlier in this chapter, peer-reviewed articles have survived the scrutiny of expert peers to ensure that the methods of data collection and analysis are sufficiently robust to yield reliable results. The first distinction readers will make, therefore, is between health texts that have or have not undergone critical scrutiny by expert peers.

Fortunately, most of the titles returned from a search of PubMed or other academic databases will draw from peer-reviewed research literature. Conversely, searching for health studies from outside academic databases usually yields synopses, news items, news summaries, or other health texts that have not received the scrutiny of impartial, expert review. These other sources of information vary in quality and trustworthiness so these should be examined with the greatest skepticism (also see Box 3.2).

BOX 3.2 GRAY LITERATURE

Gray literature encompasses a variety of health-related texts, including conference posters, abstracts, papers, graduate theses and dissertations, and data and studies reported by government agencies and private think tanks. These materials face varying degrees of scrutiny before being presented or published, leading to significant variation in their quality. For instance, articles published in the CDC's Morbidity and Mortality Weekly Report are of high quality. In contrast, a poster that reports preliminary data and is lightly reviewed for display at a conference may contain various biases and unreliable findings.

Although active seekers of high-quality evidence can easily find peer-reviewed research articles, this initial distinction remains the most essential for securing reliable evidence on which to base one's actions.

Among articles that have survived peer review, the next important distinction can be made between primary research studies and reviews of primary research studies. This is accomplished by parsing the title of the article.

Distinction 2: Primary research vs review studies

There are two major types of peer-reviewed studies found in scholarly journals – those that are *primary* research studies and those that are *reviews* of primary studies.

Primary research includes studies that collect and analyze original data or that curate and analyze "secondary" data that has already been collected. For instance, original data may be collected through questionnaires, direct observations, or experimental testing. *Secondary data* may come from administrative records, medical records, or other publicly available data (see Box 3.3).

BOX 3.3 SECONDARY DATA

Secondary data is collected for various purposes – e.g., medical records, census data, and data from online sources. Researchers will access and curate this data and prepare it for analysis. The use of secondary datasets enables access to large datasets that would not otherwise be available, saving time and resources. On the other hand, secondary data is collected for purposes that may not align with those of the researchers. There may be a mismatch in terms of inclusion of variables, validity of measures, or the level of detail the research requires. In contrast, primary data is collected under the researcher's supervision and control and, therefore, ensures alignment with the specific research need and purpose.

In contrast, review studies compare, summarize, and synthesize results from multiple primary studies on a given health issue. For instance, a systematic review of 21 primary studies found that facemasks offer significant protective effects against the flu, SARS, and COVID-19 [3]. Readers will encounter numerous types of review studies, which vary depending on the overall aim of the study – e.g., to identify research gaps, to provide a broad overview of existing literature, to aggregate statistics in a specific research area.

By inspecting the title, you can typically pigeonhole an article as describing a primary study or a review study. Often pigeonholing a review study is straightforward, as reviews would include the term "review" in the title (see Table 3.1).

In contrast, the absence of the term "review" in the title would typically indicate that the article describes a primary study. Further, since the number of primary studies far exceeds the number of review studies, most titles would indicate a primary study.

Often, the specific primary study research design is also identified in the title. Titles shown in Table 3.2 identify subtypes of primary studies, such as cross-sectional, cohort, quasi-experimental, randomized controlled trial, and qualitative studies. As you become more familiar with these types of research designs, pigeonholing them becomes easier and more specific (see Part 2).

TABLE 3.1 Pigeonholing *review* studies

#1. Efficacy of face mask in preventing respiratory virus transmission: A *systematic review* and meta-analysis [3].

#2. Mindfulness training for health profession students – *systematic review* of RCTs [4].

#3. The Mediterranean diet slows down the progression of aging and helps to prevent the onset of frailty: A *narrative review* [5].

#4. Creatine Supplementation for Muscle Growth: A *Scoping Review* of Randomized Clinical Trials from 2012 to 2021 [6].

TABLE 3.2 Pigeonholing *primary* studies

#1. Health behaviors of American pregnant women: *a cross-sectional* analysis of NHANES 2007–2014 [7].

#2. Dose-response association of aerobic and muscle-strengthening physical activity with mortality: a national *cohort* study of 416,420 US adults [8].

#3. The effect of a breastfeeding support program on breastfeeding duration and exclusivity: a *quasi-experiment* [9].

#4. The effect of green Mediterranean diet on cardiometabolic risk: a *randomised controlled trial* [10].

#5. The impact of severe asthma on patients' autonomy: A qualitative study [11].

Primary studies can be pigeonholed further based on one of two research approaches taken: quantitative or qualitative approaches.

Distinction 3: Primary studies – quantitative or qualitative

Quantitative and qualitative research offer distinct approaches to health research and differ in fundamental ways. How they differ will become more apparent in Chapters 6–11. A brief introduction to fundamental differences, however, will foster more effective pigeonholing.

Quantitative research involves using numeric data – e.g., measures of exposures and outcomes – to capture associations between exposures and health outcomes. This enhances the ability to predict or control health outcomes. For instance, a study will quantify the association between, for instance, indoor restaurant dining and testing positive for COVID-19, the Mediterranean diet and cardiovascular health, or the use of creatine supplement and athletic performance. The use of numeric data enables studies to identify factors that predict health outcomes, or the effectiveness of interventions designs to control these outcomes. In these examples, restaurant dining, the Mediterranean diet, and creating supplementation help predict various health outcomes.

In contrast, qualitative research collects non-numeric data – e.g., texts from interviews, documents, and blogs – to capture the meanings, experiences, and perspectives of human participants. This enhances mutual understanding. The qualitative framework recognizes the subjective realities of individuals, subgroups, and groups, and aims to accurately capture and represent their diverse viewpoints. For instance, qualitative studies may explore the varied experiences of pregnancy loss, nurse burnout, or caregiver support, thereby giving voice to these experiences. Whereas quantitative research attempts to predict and control phenomena, qualitative research aims to gain greater insight and understanding of human experiences and perspectives.

Given these contrasting research aims, it becomes critical for readers to distinguish between studies that take a quantitative or qualitative approach to examining the health topic.

Pigeonholing quantitative studies

Quantitative research collects and analyzes numeric data to assess the association between a health outcome and an exposure. Quantitative researchers seek to characterize relationships between variables (exposures and outcomes) – e.g., the direction (positive or negative) and strength (weak, moderate, and strong) of an association. Being able to characterize the relationship between exposure and outcome helps us predict and take actions to improve health or reduce illness.

Typically, the article's title will reveal whether the study takes a quantitative or qualitative approach, or a mixture of the two (see Table 3.3).

Certain telltale signs show these to be quantitative studies. First, each title includes terms that suggest a study of the relationship between variables. For instance, title #1 reflects a study that examined the *influences* of sedentary behavior. Title #2 examined the *effect* of community health workers on low-income patients. Title #3 examined the *impact* of ACL injury on soccer players. Titles #4 and #5 explored *relationships* and *associations*.

TABLE 3.3 Titles of *quantitative* studies

#1. Ecological Influences on Employees' Workplace Sedentary Behavior: A Cross-Sectional Study [12].
#2. Effect of Community Health Worker Support on Clinical Outcomes of Low-Income Patients Across Primary Care Facilities: A Randomized Clinical Trial [13].
#3. Impact of Anterior Cruciate Ligament Injury on European Professional Soccer Players [14].
#4. The Relationship between Food Insecurity and Esophageal and Gastric Cancers: A Case-Control Study [15].
#5. Association of cardiorespiratory fitness with long-term mortality among adults undergoing exercise treadmill testing [16].

Second, some titles will explicitly identify a type of quantitative research design used in the study. Title #1 indicates the use of a cross-sectional design; title #2 specifies the use of a randomized controlled trial; title #4 identifies the use of a case-control design.

As with any skill, pigeonholing a study as quantitative eventually becomes further refined as you come to understand observational and experimental quantitative designs (Chapters 5–9).

Pigeonholing qualitative studies

Qualitative research collects and analyzes non-numeric (text) data from various sources – interviews, online postings, documents, and field observations. Qualitative analysis aims to capture the perspectives of targeted individuals or groups, as well as the meanings they attach to various experiences. The qualitative framework recognizes that individuals and groups experience the world differently and hold different perspectives on health, illness, and healthcare. Qualitative data collection and analysis aim to characterize, understand, and gain insight into the experiences and realities of targeted individuals or groups (see Chapters 10 and 11).

Pigeonholing a qualitative study might be straightforward, as qualitative studies often include the term "qualitative" in the title. For instance,

Patient perspectives on quality of care for depression and anxiety in primary health care teams: A *qualitative* study [17].

When the term "qualitative" is not included, other terms in the title will suggest that a qualitative approach was taken. Unlike quantitative studies that focus on the relationship between exposure, intervention, and outcome, qualitative studies report the experiences, meanings, stories, and realities of people (Table 3.4).

Each title in Table 3.4 includes terms that suggest studies designed to capture the meanings and perspectives attached to experiences. Title #1 reflects a study that examined suicide *narratives*, while title #2 suggests an exploration of the *many meanings* of pregnancy loss. Titles #3 and #4 identify studies designed to capture lived *experiences* of clinicians and college students. The study identified in title #5 used *storytelling* to capture the *perspectives* of the homeless.

TABLE 3.4 Titles of *qualitative* studies

#1. Constructing and expanding suicide narratives from gay men [18].

#2. The health system and emotional care: Validating the many meanings of spontaneous pregnancy loss [19].

#3. Treatment of opioid use disorder during COVID-19: Experiences of clinicians transitioning to telemedicine [20].

#4. Examining first-generation college student lived experiences with microaggressions and microaffirmations at a predominately White public research university [21].

#5. Storytelling to capture the health care perspective of people who are homeless [22].

While these guidelines for pigeonholing studies are not fool proof, they enable readers to distinguish between quantitative and qualitative studies. As you learn more about these approaches, you will become more effective in distinguishing between them (see Chapters 5–11). Any lack of clarity that remains will be resolved as you size up the article during the next phase of inspection – reading the abstract (Chapter 4).

BOX 3.4   MIXED-METHODS STUDIES

Sometimes, qualitative and quantitative methods are combined in a single *mixed-methods* study (see Example 9.2). The two approaches can be complementary and contribute evidence on a topic. Pigeonholing a mixed-methods studies is straightforward as the terms are usually included in the title, as in: "'Ancestral recipes': a *mixed-methods* analysis of MyPlate-based recipe dissemination for Latinos in rural communities" [23].

Distinction 4: Review studies – narrative and systematic

As discussed above, article titles are often explicit about the nature of the review being conducted. There are dozens of types of review studies and no consensus on how to classify them. For current purposes, we divide review types into two types – narrative and systematic.

Briefly, traditional narrative reviews provide an overview of the state of research about a topic. In contrast, systematic reviews aim to consolidate evidence for practical decision making. A synthesis of evidence is clearest in systematic reviews that include a "meta-analysis" or "meta-synthesis".

Narrative and systematic reviews also differ with respect to their transparency regarding the methods used to locate, appraise, and analyze studies selected for review. Narrative reviews provide little or no description of the methods, whereas systematic reviews are fully transparent in describing the methods for the review (see Chapter 12).

In view of their fundamental differences, one can readily distinguish between traditional narrative and systematic reviews by the title. As suggested in Table 3.1, systematic reviews almost always include the term "systematic review" in the title – e.g., Efficacy of face mask in preventing respiratory virus transmission: A *systematic review* and meta-analysis [3]. Though less common, narrative reviews will also include the term "narrative" in the title. Often, narrative reviews can be identified by a less structured abstract and little to no reference to the methods used to select, appraise, and analyze the studies under review.

The various distinctions made when pigeonholing an article's title help identify the *type* of study the article describes. Based on the type of study, readers will gain insight into the nature and type of findings the study will provide. As discussed below, the title is also rich in information about the content of the study – the health topic of the study explored.

Pigeonholing the title by *topic*

Titles of peer-reviewed articles tell us more than the type of study being described and the nature of the findings a study will supply. Titles, of course, provide information about the content of the study and the specific topic being explored. Thus, parsing titles also gives the reader a clearer idea about topical aspects of the study – e.g., the sample population, health outcomes, exposures, or experiences. As shown in Table 3.5, titles are often rich in information about the content of the study.

All the titles would be pigeonholed as primary studies – experimental, cross-sectional, and qualitative. The titles also provide readers information about the content of the article, enabling articles to be screened for relevance to the health topic. Parsing the title for topic-related information yields additional information about the study and its relevance to the reader.

For instance, by parsing title #1, readers identify the study design, sample population, and key variables – a cross-sectional study of the health behaviors of pregnant American women. For title #2, an experiment was conducted with young adults to test the effects of an intervention on anxiety. For title #3, a qualitative study was conducted to capture the experience of physical therapy among patients with low back pain.

TABLE 3.5 Pigeonholing by topic-related information

Title and topic-related information
#1. Health behaviors of American pregnant women: a cross-sectional analysis of NHANES 2007–2014 [7] • Study *design*: cross-sectional • Sample *population*: American pregnant women. • Key *variables*: health behaviors
#2. Differential experimental effects of a short bout of walking, meditation, or combination of walking and meditation on state anxiety among young adults [24]. • Study *design*: experimental • Sample *population*: young adults • Key *variables*: meditation/walking interventions (intervention); state anxiety (outcome)
#3. Beyond the pain: A qualitative study exploring the physical therapy experience in patients with chronic low back pain [25]. • Study design: qualitative • Sample population: patients with chronic low back pain • Key qualitative issue: physical therapy experience

It almost goes without saying that titles should be carefully read. The study may or may not align with your reading aim, but the issue is often settled in short order by carefully inspecting the title. Where uncertainty remains, readers will turn to the summary description of the study as presented in the article's abstract.

Recap

This chapter discussed the inspectional stage of reading, the essential first step in assessing the relevance of studies returned from a search. This stage involves parsing an article's title to "pigeonhole" it by its type – e.g., peer-reviewed, primary research, review study, and quantitative or qualitative study. It also involves identifying key components of the health topic in the title – e.g., the health outcomes, exposures, and study population – readers gain additional insight into the article's relevance.

The chapter also suggests that it is worth the short time it takes to pigeonhole the title by type and topic in that it enables the exclusion of most titles as irrelevant to the reader's purpose, while helping to focus the inquiry. As discussed in the next chapter, the remaining studies will be further scrutinized by inspecting the abstract.

References

1. Institute of Medicine. *To err is human: Building a safer health system.* Washington, DC: National Academy Press; 2000.
2. Institute of Medicine. *Crossing the quality chasm: A new health system for the 21st century.* Washington, DC: National Academy Press; 2001.
3. Liang M, Gao L, Cheng C, Zhou Q, Uy JP, Heiner K, Sun C. Efficacy of face mask in preventing respiratory virus transmission: A systematic review and meta-analysis. *Travel Med Infect Dis.* 2020;36(March): 101751. doi:10.1016/j.tmaid.2020.101751.
4. McConville J, McAleer R, Hahne A. Mindfulness training for health profession students— systematic review of RCTs. *Explore (NY).* 2017;13(1):26–45. doi:10.1097/BRS.0b013e 3182a7f449.
5. Capurso C, Bellanti F, Buglio AL, Vendemiale G. The Mediterranean diet slows down the progression of aging and helps to prevent the onset of frailty: A narrative review. *Nutrients.* 2020;12(1). doi:10.3390/nu12010035.
6. Wu SH, Chen KL, Hsu C, Chen HC, Chen JY, Yu SY, Shiu YJ. Creatine supplementation for muscle growth: A scoping review of randomized clinical trials from 2012 to 2021. *Nutrients.* 2022;14(6):35. doi:10.3390/nu14061255.
7. Francis EC, Zhang L, Witrick B, Chen L. Health behaviors of American pregnant women: A cross-sectional analysis of NHANES 2007-2014. *J Public Health (Oxf).* 2021;43(1):131–138. doi:10.1093/pubmed/fdz117.
8. Coleman CJ, McDonough DJ, Pope ZC, Pope CA. Dose-response association of aerobic and muscle-strengthening physical activity with mortality: A national cohort study of 416,420 US adults. *Br J Sports Med.* 2022: bjsports-2022-105519. doi:10.1136/bjsports-2021-104567.
9. van Dellen SA, Wisse B, Mobach MP, Dijkstra A. The effect of a breastfeeding support programme on breastfeeding duration and exclusivity: A quasi-experiment. *BMC Public Health.* 2019;19(1):993. doi:10.1186/s12889-019-7331-y.
10. Tsaban G, Meir AY, Rinott E, Zelicha H, Kaplan A, Shalev A, et al. The effect of green Mediterranean diet on cardiometabolic risk; A randomised controlled trial. *Heart.* 2021;107(13):1054–1061. doi:10.1136/heartjnl-2020-317802.
11. Eassey D, Reddel HK, Ryan K, Smith L. The impact of severe asthma on patients' autonomy: A qualitative study. *Health Expect.* 2019;22(3):528–536. doi:10.1111/hex.12879.

12. Wilkerson AH, Usdan SL, Knowlden AP, Leeper JL, Birch DA, Hibberd EE. Ecological influences on employees' workplace sedentary behavior: A cross-sectional study. *Am J Health Promot.* 2018; 32(8):1688–1696. doi:10.1177/0890117118767717.
13. Kangovi S, Mitra N, Norton L, Harte R, Zhao X, Carter T, et al. Effect of community health worker support on clinical outcomes of low-income patients across primary care facilities: A randomized clinical trial. *JAMA Intern Med.* 2018;178(12):1635–1643. doi:10.1001/jamainternmed.2018.4630.
14. Mazza D, Viglietta E, Monaco E, Iorio R, Marzilli F, Princi G, et al. Impact of anterior cruciate ligament injury on European professional soccer players. *Orthop J Sports Med.* 2022;10(2). doi:10.1177/23259671221076865.
15. Daneshi-Maskooni M, Badri-Fariman M, Habibi N, Dorosty-Motlagh A, Yavari H, Kashani A, et al. The relationship between food insecurity and esophageal and gastric cancers: A case-control study. *J Res Health Sci.* 2017;17(2):e00381.
16. Mandsager K, Harb S, Cremer P, Phelan D, Nissen SE, Jaber W. Association of cardiorespiratory fitness with long-term mortality among adults undergoing exercise treadmill testing. *JAMA Netw Open.* 2018;1(6):e183605. doi:10.1001/jamanetworkopen.2018.3605.
17. Ashcroft R, Menear M, Greenblatt A, Silveira J, Dahrouge S, Sunderji N, et al. Patient perspectives on quality of care for depression and anxiety in primary health care teams: A qualitative study. *Health Expect.* 2021;24(4):1168–1177. doi:10.1111/hex.13242.
18. Salway T, Gesink D. Constructing and expanding suicide narratives from gay men. *Qual Health Res.* 2018;28(11):1788–1801. doi:10.1177/1049732318782432.
19. Corbet-Owen C, Kruger LM. The health system and emotional care: Validating the many meanings of spontaneous pregnancy loss. *Fam Syst Health.* 2001;19(4):411–427. doi:10.1037/h0089469.
20. Uscher-Pines L, Sousa J, Raja P, Mehrotra A, Barnett M, Huskamp HA. Treatment of opioid use disorder during COVID-19: Experiences of clinicians transitioning to telemedicine. *J Subst Abuse Treat.* 2020;118:108124. doi:10.1016/j.jsat.2020.108124.
21. Ellis JM, Powell CS, Demetriou CP, Huerta-Bapat C, Panter AT. Examining first-generation college student lived experiences with microaggressions and microaffirmations at a predominately white public research university. *Cultur Divers Ethnic Minor Psychol.* 2019;25(2):266–279. doi:10.1037/cdp0000198.
22. Moore-Nadler M, Clanton C, Roussel L. Storytelling to capture the health care perspective of people who are homeless. *Qual Health Res.* 2019. doi:10.1177/1049732319857058.
23. Cheney AM, McCarthy WJ, Pozar M, Reaves C, Ortiz G, Lopez D, et al. "Ancestral recipes": A mixed-methods analysis of MyPlate-based recipe dissemination for Latinos in rural communities. *BMC Public Health.* 2023;23:216. doi:10.1186/s12889-022-14804-3.
24. Edwards MK, Rosenbaum S, Loprinzi PD. Differential experimental effects of a short bout of walking, meditation, or combination of walking and meditation on state anxiety among young adults. *Am J Health Promot.* 2018;32(4):949–958. doi:10.1177/0890117117744913.
25. Joyce C, Keysor J, Stevans J, Ready K, Roseen EJ, Saper RB. Beyond the pain: A qualitative study exploring the physical therapy experience in patients with chronic low back pain. *Physiother Theory Pract.* 2023;39(4):803–813. doi:10.1080/09593985.2022.2029650.

4

INSPECTION 2

Assessing an article's relevance

Overview: sizing up the article

Inspecting an article involves two steps. The first – pigeonholing and parsing the title – was discussed in Chapter 3. Parsing the title is the quickest way to exclude articles from consideration. Articles that remain involve the second inspectional phase – reading the abstract. The abstract provides a summary description of the study – the aim, methods, results, and conclusions. This summary description will inform the decision about whether to critically analyze the study's full text to gain a deeper understanding of the findings and their implications for evidence-based practice.

Dissecting the abstract

Most titles contain between 10 and 20 words, whereas an abstract expands to 250 or so, depending on the journal. Abstracts contain the basic storyline of the article. Abstracts outline four key ingredients of the study in this order

1 the aim or purpose of the study
2 methods of data collection and analysis – e.g., sample and design
3 major findings – e.g., statistics and themes
4 major conclusions

The abstract offers a concise summary of each of these major components.

The study's aim

The first component of a study's storyline involves the study's aim or purpose. This appears as the initial sentence or passage of the abstract. For instance, in a study on the

DOI: 10.4324/9781003595663-5

effects of meditation and walking on anxiety, the aim is presented in the abstract under the label "Introduction":

> **Introduction**: Single bouts of aerobic exercise and meditation have been shown to improve anxiety states. Yet to be evaluated in the literature, we sought to examine the effects of a single, short bout of aerobic exercise or meditation, as well as exercise and meditation combined on state anxiety among young adults [1].

This passage includes a brief rationale for undertaking the study. In this case, the aim – to examine the "anxiolytic" effects of short bouts of walking and medication – is accompanied by a short statement that suggests the need for the study – these effects have not yet been evaluated. The Introduction section in the body of the article elaborates further on the current evidence, research need, and the study's aim.

Methods – participants, design, analysis

The next component of the article's storyline is the methods used to achieve this aim. The methods are defined by the key features of the data collection and analysis process. In the abstract, this usually involves a brief description of the study participants, the research design, the key variables, and the analysis.

Abstracts may outline the methods in somewhat different ways. This one is more detailed than most, specifying four components of the methods – the design, setting, study subjects, and measures [1]:

> **Design**: Randomized controlled trial.
> **Setting**: University.
> **Subjects**: Participants ($N = 110$, mean age = 21.4 years) were randomly assigned to walk, meditate, walk then meditate, meditate then walk, or to sit (inactive control).
> **Measures**: All walking and meditation bouts were 10 minutes in duration. Participants' state anxiety was monitored before and after the intervention using the State Trait Anxiety Inventory questionnaire.

The design and setting are simply identified – a randomized control trial (RCT) was carried out in a university setting (Chapters 10 and 11). RCTs are a specific type of experimental design where subjects are randomly assigned to groups and are commonly found in health science research (see Chapter 8). The University is a familiar setting that traditionally include mainly young adults, in this case with an average age of 21.4 years. The treatment intervention used in the RCT was described in terms of 10-minute bouts of walking and meditation; the health outcome was measured using the "State-Trait Anxiety Inventory". These various components of the methods are not always included as they are here, but this example illustrates several you might find in an abstract.

Results

From the methods used to collect and analyze data come the results. This portion of the abstract highlights the key findings from the study

> **Results:** Significant group X time interaction effects were observed ($p = .01$). Post hoc paired t tests revealed that state anxiety significantly decreased from baseline to postintervention in the meditation ($p = .002$), meditation then walk ($p = .002$), and walk then meditation ($p = .03$) groups but not the walk ($p = .75$) or control ($p = .45$) groups.

Health professionals with different levels of training and experience will variously understand the statistical procedures used (e.g., group X time effects, paired t-tests). Even without knowing (yet) what post hoc t-tests are, readers can surmise from the abstract that anxiety declined from baseline to post-intervention for different groups. Moreover, based on the "p-values", this relationship was "statistically significant" – i.e., the findings suggest an association between meditation and anxiety.

Conclusion

The conclusion offers the author's interpretation of what the results mean – their implications for future research, health practice, or health policy:

> **Conclusion:** Meditation (versus a brisk walk) may be a preferred method of attenuating anxiety symptomology. Individuals desiring the health benefits associated with aerobic exercise may achieve additional anxiolytic benefits if they employ a brief meditation session before or after exercising.

Here, the conclusion remains close to what the results tell us but offers practical advice to individuals who wish to reduce their anxiety – even brief meditation (or meditation plus walking) provides anxiolytic benefits.

From the title and abstract, you will obtain a summary of the study and its overall conclusions. This may be sufficient for decisions of lesser risk or for immediate purposes. Yet the findings and conclusions of a study must be taken at face value and without any critical scrutiny. Thus, relying solely on the evidence presented in the abstract can lead to a partial understanding, potentially leading to ineffective or harmful practice decisions. A more crucial role of the abstract is to help one decide whether a critical examination of the article is needed to gain a deeper understanding of the quality and limitations of the results and their application to evidence-based practice.

Discerning the article's relevance

The purpose of inspectional reading is to gather enough information about the type and topic of the study to gauge whether it deserves further analytical reading. Foremost, this depends on the study's alignment with the reader's objective. As shown in Figure 4.1,

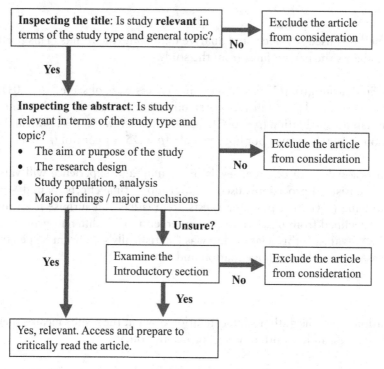

FIGURE 4.1 A flowchart – the process of inspecting the title and abstract of an article in order to determine its relevance to the reading aim.

some key decision points are available during inspection for readers to assess this alignment and potentially advance to reading the article analytically.

1 **Inspecting the title.** From the title, readers learn about the type and topic of study and will assess its alignment with their aim or purpose. Many articles are first excluded based on pigeonholing and parsing the title.
2 **Inspecting the abstract.** The abstract summarizes the main components of the study – background, methods, results, conclusions. From this summary information readers will learn more about key components of the study and revisit the decision concerning its relevance. Studies deemed not relevant are excluded. The full text of relevant studies is accessed for analytical reading.
3 **Examine the Introduction.** If uncertainty regarding the relevance of a study remains after examining the abstract, readers may then turn their attention to the introductory section in the body of the article. As described below, the Introduction will provide the rationale underlying the study, and a clearer picture of the study's main hypotheses or objectives. With this additional background, readers can gauge an article's alignment with their reading objective, and whether to exclude the article, or retain it for analytical reading.

Articles accessed and retained for analytical reading might be skimmed to identify the headings and subheadings, and tables and figures to be encountered. It also provides a picture of the overall structure of the article.

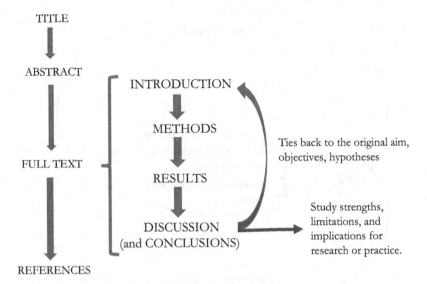

FIGURE 4.2 The structure of the typical research article.

Understanding the structure of a research article

With some variation, you can expect the body of the article to be structured like the abstract is structured. Most research articles roughly divide into four sections: (1) the Introduction (or Background) section, (2) the Methods section, (3) the Results section, and (4) the Discussion and Conclusion (see Figure 4.2).

There are divisions and subdivisions of each of the four major sections, but each division contributes something to the overall logic of the research study and article.

The introduction

The introductory section serves as a bridge between inspectional and analytical reading. It provides the rationale for conducting the study, which may inform both the decision to critically examine the methods, results, and the background evidence placing the study in a larger research context.

As shown in Figure 4.3, the Introduction divides into four parts, each providing a background information and, taken together, offering a rationale for the study

1 the general topic of the study;
2 the research surrounding the topic;
3 the research gap (in our knowledge about the topic);
4 the research need and study objectives.

The general topic

The general topic is already known from inspectional reading but is further described in the opening of the article. This description often starts with a claim about the importance of studying the topic. For instance, a study of health behaviors among American

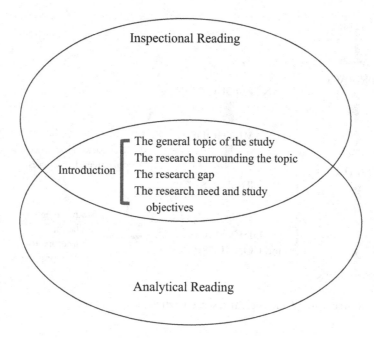

The general topic of the study
The research surrounding the topic
The research gap
The research need and study objectives

Introduction

Inspectional Reading

Analytical Reading

FIGURE 4.3 The introduction – bridging inspectional and analytical reading.

pregnant women opens with: "From a life-course perspective, the prenatal period has been recognized as a critical period for both women and their offspring" [2]. The references at the end of the opener point the reader toward evidence to support their claim.

The surrounding research

The Introductory section describes the research context from which the specific study objectives arise. The surrounding research includes the various theories and findings from recent studies that relate to the topic. This can be viewed as a mini-literature review where findings from key studies are described. The in-text citations serve to embed the current study within the surrounding research.

For instance, three citations connect a single assertion in a study about health behaviors of pregnant women

Physical activity and adequate sleep have been recognized as important health behaviors to protect against pregnancy complications such as gestational diabetes, which increases women's risk of later developing type II diabetes. [2]

In this example, the study identifies specific health behaviors – physical activity and sleep – as important for reducing complications (type II diabetes) during and after pregnancy. Over 20 in-text citations connected the current study to others describing the effects of vitamins, physical activity, sleep, smoking and diet on pregnancy and birth. Citations in the Introduction section define the context of the current study.

The research gap

After describing the theory and evidence surrounding the topic, the Introduction identifies the limits of the research – what is *not* yet known about the topic. Again, in the study of pregnancy behaviors, the Introduction identifies a limitation of the evidence the studies provide

> Although the importance of health behaviors during pregnancy has been acknowledged by various professional organizations, the proportion of US women who engage in several recommended health behaviors is not clear.
>
> [2]

In other words, while we understand that healthy behaviors during pregnancy are important for infants and women, it remains unclear to what degree do groups of American women adhere to recommended practices.

The research need and study objectives

This limit to our understanding suggests a research need that should be filled. This research need underlies the objectives of the study. For instance, since the proportion of women who engage in the recommended behaviors is unclear, the objective of the study was to…

> … examine engagement in five recommended health behaviors (adequate fruit and vegetable consumption, prenatal multivitamin use, adequate physical activity, adequate sleep and abstention from smoking).
>
> [2]

The study objectives define the direction of the study, shaping the methods used to collect and analyze data, and the results that follow (Box 4.1).

BOX 4.1   RESEARCH OBJECTIVES

Research objectives might also be expressed as a research aim, purpose, question, or hypothesis. Either way, they serve to focus the study. Research aims are broadly defined in the abstract, but they are more clearly specified as objectives at the end of the Introductory section.

The Introduction serves as a mini-literature review of the theory and evidence surrounding a health topic, and this review provides the context and rationale for the study objectives. Although the content of introductory sections varies from study to study, the overall logic of the section is similar across research articles.

Knowing and understanding this logic enables readers to examine subsections of the Introduction that are relevant to them, even if only to skim through them. The specific objectives of the study are important for showing readers the overall direction of the study as well as to allow readers to revisit the question of relevance.

The methods and results

The next two sections of research articles describe study methods and the results of these methods. The two are inextricably linked, although the results always depend on the methods used to produce them (not vice-versa). Thus, to understand the results, it is important to understand the methods used to produce them.

The Methods section describes the research design, which serves as a blueprint for data collection and analysis. The Methods section describes where and from whom data were collected, how observations were made, and the tools used to record them (e.g., instrumentation, questionnaires, interviews, recording devices). The Methods also describe how the data are analyzed – the procedures used to transform raw data into the findings reported in the Results section.

While the Methods describes the research plan, the Results section describes the fruits of the plan. For quantitative studies, findings are presented as statistics that characterize the nature and strength of the relationships observed in the sample population. They are shown in tables, charts, figures, and in surrounding text. For non-numeric data collected in qualitative studies, findings are typically described in terms of broader themes to characterize the experiences and perspectives of research subjects and are often supplemented with quotes from study participants.

Although the results are usually the reader's chief interest, to read critically and analytically requires reading and understanding the methods used to produce them. Results are always partial and limited, and sometimes highly skewed and unreliable. Taking them at face value, misinterpreting them, and misapplying them can lead to outcomes that are ineffective, harmful, or potentially dangerous. The transparency of scientific research allows anyone to critically assess findings and conclusions. As discussed in Parts 2 and 3, analytic questions will guide the process of critically reading and analyzing the methods and results.

Discussion (and conclusion)

The fourth major section in an article is the Discussion section. The section discusses the study results, describing how they compare with other studies, and the study's contribution to our understanding of the issue. Importantly, it also discusses the study's limitations – how certain biases might distort the results, or areas where the results may not apply. Articles conclude by suggesting some implications of the study for health research or practice.

Recap

This chapter described how to assess articles that have passed the initial title inspection by examining the abstract. It described the main components of the abstract – the aim, methods, key findings, and conclusions. It suggested that by inspecting the abstract, readers will gain valuable information about the study's aim(s), participants, methods of data collection and analysis, and key findings. Examining the abstract helps to inform decisions about whether to go deeper into a critical examination of the full text of the article.

Finally, the Chapter described the essential structure of a research article, one that resembles a structured abstract. The body of an article includes (1) an introduction that provides an overview of the evidence that serves as background to the study, (2) the methods used to collect and analyze data, (3) study results, and (4) a discussion of the study's strengths, limitations, and implications.

References

1. Edwards MK, Rosenbaum S, Loprinzi PD. Differential experimental effects of a short bout of walking, meditation, or combination of walking and meditation on state anxiety among young adults. *Am J Health Promot*. 2018;32(4):949–958. doi:10.1177/0890117117744913.
2. Francis EC, Zhang L, Witrick B, Chen L. Health behaviors of American pregnant women: A cross-sectional analysis of NHANES 2007–2014. *J Public Health (Oxf)*. 2021;43(1):131–138. https://doi.org/10.1093/pubmed/fdz117.

PART 2

Analytically reading primary studies

Part 1 of this text emphasizes the importance of inspecting titles and abstracts to grasp the fundamental aim, methods, results, and conclusions of a study. Inspection offers a way to help gauge the study's relevance to the reader and to determine whether a study deserves a deeper, analytical reading.

Part 2 is about critically analyzing primary studies and the findings they report (Chapters 5–11). Analytically reading primary studies involves asking questions of the studies and transparency requires clear answers in return. Chapter 5 identifies ten (10) questions to use to analytically read quantitative studies.

Chapters 6–9 cover two types of quantitative designs – observational and experimental. Chapter 6 provides a conceptual overview of three subtypes of observational designs – cross-sectional, case-control, and cohort designs. To show how the 10 questions may be applied to critically analyze these studies, Chapter 7 provides four examples of studies that use observational designs. Similarly, Chapter 8 provides a conceptual overview of three experimental designs – natural- quasi- and true- experimental designs, and Chapter 9 provides examples experimental studies using the 10 questions to critically examine them.

Finally, Chapter 10 provides an overview of qualitative studies as whole. Qualitative research differs fundamentally from quantitative research. Correspondingly, the questions used to analyze the methods and results of qualitative studies differ. These analytical questions are also discussed in Chapter 10. Chapter 11 then shows how these questions can be employed to analyze two qualitative studies.

DOI: 10.4324/9781003595663-6

5

TEN (10) QUESTIONS FOR ANALYTICALLY READING QUANTITATIVE STUDIES

Overview – analytically reading quantitative studies

As Part 1 discussed, inspecting an article enables the reader to learn what the study is about, its objectives, methods, and key findings. Inspection provides an overview of the study but offers little in regarding how and where findings might apply. Inspectional reading primarily informs decisions about a study's potential relevance to the reader's aim and whether the study and its findings deserve more in-depth analysis.

Analytical reading involves the active examination of the full text of the article, asking questions of it, and expecting answers in return. These questions inquire about what the findings indicate, how they were generated, and how and where they apply. The transparency of research articles is, of course, necessary for answering these questions.

Asking questions activates the reading process. The questions direct the reader in examining the text. The text is not passively received, but actively interrogated. Asking questions empowers the student and health professional with a broader and deeper understanding of the evidence that informs health decisions.

Table 5.1 includes ten (10) questions that the reader can ask of a quantitative study. (Chapters 10 and 13 identify questions to be asked of qualitative studies and systematic reviews.) The questions are associated with each of the four major sections of the article.

The questions are broad enough to cover the four main sections outlined in Chapter 4. The first two are addressed during inspectional reading (Q1 and Q2). The question about study design, initially answered in the title or the abstract, is fleshed out in the Methods section (Q3–Q5). These questions address the process of data collection (sampling and variable measurement) and (statistical) analysis.

The questions for the Methods section set the stage for the critical examination of study's results (Q6–Q8). The questions ask about the results of data collection and analysis – findings about the sample and the relationship between health outcomes and exposures. Readers will use what they learned about the methods of data collection and analysis to evaluate these findings.

DOI: 10.4324/9781003595663-7

TABLE 5.1 Ten (10) questions for analytically reading quantitative studies

Section	Question
Title, Abstract, Introduction	Q1 Is the study relevant?
	Q2 What study design was used?
Methods	Q3 What inclusion/ exclusion criteria did the study use to select the sample?
	Q4 How valid and reliable were the variable measures?
	Q5 How were the data analyzed?
Results	Q6 How was the sample characterized?
	Q7 Which relationships were reported to be statistically significant (or not)?
	Q8 How strong were the relationships?
Discussion and Conclusion	Q9 What were the strengths and limitations of the study?
	Q10 What were the implications of the study for research and practice?

Finally, questions Q9 and Q10 ask about the contributions and limitations of the study, as well as the implications of the results for research and practice. Readers will necessarily interpret the study and its findings when evaluating how they apply to health decisions.

What follows elaborates on how these questions will assist in analytically reading quantitative studies.

Inspection and the introduction – Q1 and Q2

Typically, the first two questions readers are answered by inspecting the article's title and abstract:

Q1. Is the study relevant (to your current aims)?
Q2. What study design was used?

How relevant a study is with respect to your current aim is probably the most basic and important question to ask of any article. Reading articles that appear "interesting" can address some curiosity but does little to inform evidence-based practice. The answer to Q1 often comes from the title itself, or the title and abstract. It may be firmed up while skimming the introductory section and finding compelling research needs and clear study objectives. The answer becomes easier the clearer your own aims become – when you know better the type and quality of study you are looking for.

Through inspection one pigeonholes a study by its type – a review study (traditional narrative or systematic), a quantitative study (observational or experimental), or a qualitative study. The study's research design reflects this. The type or design of the study lets you know what the study might give you in terms of evidence. The more familiar you become with different research designs, the easier it becomes to recognize study designs along with the results they yield. In turn, this can have implications for decisions concerning the study's relevance.

Knowing the framework of the research design helps readers understand how different components of the methods fit together. These components are described more fully in the Methods section.

The methods section – Q3, Q4, and Q5

Q3   What inclusion/exclusion criteria did the study use to select the sample?

Articles describe who or what subjects would be eligible for inclusion in the study. For instance, a quasi-experiment designed to test the effects of a breastfeeding support program specified as the inclusion criteria

(1) being pregnant; (2) planning to breastfeed; (3) having access to the internet; (4) having singleton gestation; (5) non-missing data for breastfeeding duration [1].

The source of research subjects is identified in this section and should be noted. In this example, the source of the support program is a Dutch health insurance company, so pregnant women outside this program would be excluded. It is natural to ask whether pregnant women from the Netherlands would respond to the support program in the same way women from other nations would. And if not, it is reasonable to ask how they differ and what program adjustments might be made to adapt the intervention for pregnant women from different populations.

Further, not everyone who is eligible necessarily participates in the study. How the sample of eligible participants is chosen may skew the sample toward certain groups or individuals and, thereby, affect the results. *Selection bias* often occurs when non-random procedures determine who participates in the study (Box 5.1 and Appendix B). For instance, research participants may be secured through referrals from physicians or other health professionals. This opens the question of bias and whether referrals favor some subjects over others – e.g., healthier subjects, those expected to respond well to a treatment.

Readers should be aware of possible selection bias in studies that rely on volunteers for study participants. For instance, a study of health behaviors that relies on readily available volunteers might attract a disproportionate number of health-conscious and capable individuals to the study. Study results might apply to eager volunteers but not to the "average" group or individual. Who is likely to volunteer may depend on various factors such as gender, age, race, availability, or perceived relevance.

In short, what naturally follows from learning what eligibility criteria are used is an evaluation of how study participants resemble or differ from the individuals the health professional is targeting and, therefore, how and where the study results might apply.

BOX 5.1   RANDOM *SAMPLING* AND RANDOM *ASSIGNMENT*

Random *sampling* is used to limit biases in the selection of study participants. Unlike convenience sampling or reliance on volunteers, with random sampling everyone included in the study population has an equal chance of being selected. Random sampling should not be confused with random *assignment*. Random sampling involves selecting research subjects from a larger study population. Random assignment involves assigning participants to experimental groups randomly. Thus, random assignment occurs after the sampling process (see Chapter 8).

Q4 How valid and reliable were the variable measures?

A fundamental aspect of the data collection process is the measurement of variables in the study – e.g., the health outcome, exposure, and covariates. Variable measures quantify observations. A description of variable measures usually follows the discussion of the study population. Analytical reading involves asking how observations translate into measures and the reliability and validity of these measures.

Reliability and validity

In quantitative studies, abstract concepts are defined and operationalized as variable measures – a set of numbers designed to reflect specific values of observations. For instance, the concept of gender might be recorded as "1" (female), "2" (male), and "3" (other). Adult age might be measured in years ranging from 18 to 100.

Any concept can be measured, all with varying degrees of reliability (consistency) and validity (accuracy). Automated blood pressure monitors may more reliably measure blood pressure than, say, an untrained person using a stethoscope and blood pressure cuff. A structured interview with a health professional will provide a more reliable measure of depression than, say, respondents' self-reports of their overall mood.

Some variable measures may be more valid than others as well. An accelerometer provides a more valid measure of physical activity than self-reports of physical activity, which are subject to *self-report bias* (see Appendix B) – respondents imperfectly recall past physical activities (recall bias), or they may over-state their physical activity to present themselves in a favorable light (social desirability).

Readers should be alert to the reliability and validity of variable measures, particularly measures of the health outcome and prior exposure. Newly constructed measures, while suitable for a given study, have not been assessed in terms of their reliability and validity. Consequently, readers would rely on the "face validity" of these measures – how the measures appear on their service – to gauge their accuracy.

In contrast, studies more often use measures that have been tested for reliability and validity and also will include citations to these tests. Some variable measures are so widely known and used that they appear as the standard in a research area. These bring confidence to assessments of the validity of the findings. Moreover, results produced by commonly used measurements can be compared with results from other studies. Such comparisons foster the accumulation of evidence and the refinement of theories.

Q5 How were the data analyzed?

Numeric data allow for statistical analysis designed to describe the sample population and to characterize relationships among variables – e.g., health outcomes and exposures). Statistical analyses allow relationships between variables to be characterized in terms of their statistical significance (Appendix D and Appendix E) and strength of association or effect size (Appendix F).

Statistical significance

Quantitative studies rely on numerous statistical operations to analyze numeric data. Fundamentally, these methods include statistical tests to determine whether a relationship is "statistically significant". A relationship is deemed as statistically significant if the observed association between two variables is unlikely to have occurred by chance or random coincidence. Findings that cannot be explained by chance are seen as supporting the alternative explanation for this significant relationship (see Box 5.2).

Health researchers use the "p-value" to set a threshold to gauge whether a relationship is "statistically significant" (see Appendix D). This threshold or *alpha level* for statistical significance is commonly set to $\alpha \leq 0.05$. Relationships where the p-value falls at or below 0.05 would be considered as statistically significant. The Results section of the article will identify which relationships are statistically significant and which ones are not.

BOX 5.2 NULL AND ALTERNATIVE HYPOTHESES

The p-value is an outcome of a test of the "null" hypothesis. The null or default hypothesis is that there is no association between variables (e.g., outcomes, exposures, and interventions). The alternative research hypothesis is that there are significant differences and effects. A low p-value indicates a low chance that the default or null hypothesis is true – e.g., ≤ 0.05. The null hypothesis would be rejected in favor of the alternative or research hypothesis. Thus, a low p-value provides evidence that supports an alternative hypothesis.

Strength of association or effect size

A relationship might be statistically significant but not very strong or of little or no concern when it comes to practical decisions. That is why it is also important for readers to assess the strength of the relationship between exposure and outcome or the size of the effect of an intervention on an outcome.

Studies use different metrics to capture the strength of an association or the size of an effect. For instance, a new dietary intervention might produce an average weight loss of 10 pounds. Another intervention might reduce weight by 5 pounds. The effect size is easy to see and interpret and is measured in absolute terms – an average weight loss of 10 pounds in one intervention and 5 pounds in the other.

Statistical measures that express the strength of an association in relative terms are less straightforward and require additional interpretation. For instance, in the dietary intervention example discussed above, a comparative measure such as an odds ratio might suggest that one diet is, on average, twice as effective for weight loss compared to the other. The odds ratio (OR) would be OR = 2.0. To fully grasp the implications of these numbers, readers often translate these coefficients into meaningful terms.

The Pearson correlation coefficient (the Pearson *r*) measures the strength and direction of the association between two numeric variables – how variation in one variable correlates with variation in another variable. As shown in Figure 5.1, the strength of the Pearson *r* is indicated by how tightly clustered the data points are around a trend line cuts through the middle of the spread – the more tightly clustered the data points are around the trend line, the greater the value of Pearson *r*.

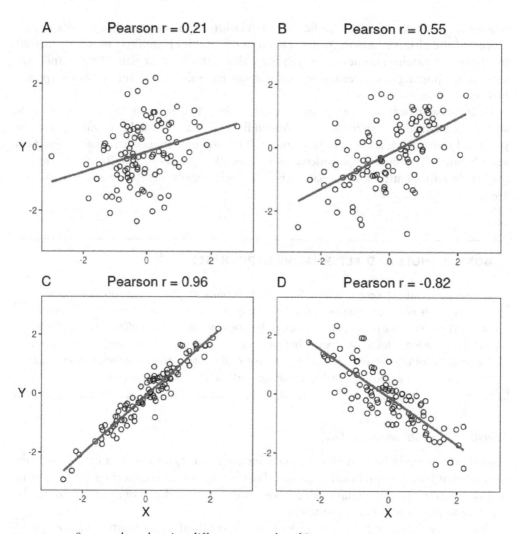

FIGURE 5.1 Scatter plots showing different strengths of Pearson r.

Each dot on a scatterplot represents a case and the case is defined by the value on X and Y variables. For instance, in plot A, cases are scattered every which way and the Pearson r = low ($r = 0.21$). Knowing the value of X would be of little help for predicting the value of Y. Plot B shows a moderate association ($r = 0.55$). Cases in plot C are tightly clustered around the trend line – the more tightly clustered, the greater the correlation ($r = 0.96$) – knowing a case's value on X would be of considerable help in estimating the value on Y.

Pearson r also characterizes the direction of the relationship. For instance, aerobic activity and lung function would correlate positively – higher aerobic activity would be associated with higher lung function. Cigarette smoking and lung function might vary negatively, however, where higher smoking levels is associated with lower lung function. Plot D shows a negative association – as the value of X increases, the value of Y decreases ($r = -0.82$).

TABLE 5.2 Examples of effect size statistics and their interpretation

Statistic	Rule-of-thumb Interpretation
OR, RR, and HR	1.0 means no difference between two groups.
ranges from 0.0 to infinity	to infinity = increasing difference favoring one group
(two binary variables)	1.0 to 0.0 = increasing difference favoring the other groups
Cohen's d*	d = circa 0.20 is a "small" difference between means
Ranges from 0.0 to infinity (one	d = circa 0.50 is "moderate" between means
binary, one numeric variable)	d = circa 0.80 or greater is "large" difference between means
Pearson r	r = 0.00 to ± 0.30 is a "small" correlation between two
Ranges from −1.0 to 1.0 (two	variables
numeric variables)	r = ±0.30 to ± 0.70 is "medium" correlation between two variables
	r = ≥ 0.70 or ≤ −0.70 is "large" correlation between two variables

* Mean differences compare differences between groups or differences before and after an intervention.

Pearson r characterizes the strength and direction of the relationship between two continuous or numeric variables (e.g., height and weight, exercise, and lung function). Cohen's d quantifies the average change (effect size) that occurs between experimental groups (see Table 5.2 and Appendix F). For instance, one might compare the change that occurs between groups undergoing different physical training regimes to see the relative effects on cardiovascular fitness. The average improvement in cardiovascular fitness may be one standard deviation greater for group A compared to group B.

Other commonly used measures of association are odds, risk, and hazard ratios – ORs, RRs, and HRs. As ratios, they quantify the strength of the association between two binary or dichotomous variables. A binary or dichotomous variable is a type of variable that can only take on two possible values – e.g., "Yes or No", "either-or", "present or absent", and "0 or 1" variable. The ratios compare exposures (i.e., present-absent) to health outcomes (i.e., present-absent). For instance, one might compare the ratio of people who have or have not been exposed to a smoking cessation program in terms of whether they did or did not quit smoking – e.g., cessation might be 3.2 times (OR=3.2) more likely among those who experienced the program compared to those who did not (Appendix F).

It is often challenging to translate the quantity expressed in a statistic into terms that have clear meaning to the reader. Occasionally, studies will translate these quantities into more tangible and meaningful units. For instance, one study translated the effect of raising the minimum wage on depression – a 0.37 standard deviation in improvement – to about the equivalent to the "effect size estimated for antidepressants ... on depressive symptoms" [2]. For these general statistics, certain "rules of thumb" may be used to translate numerical values into meaningful interpretations.

These statistics are meant to capture the strength of an association between variables. Analytical reading involves assessing not only whether the relationship is "statistically significant", but also how strong that relationship is. Stronger relationships will generally be more practically meaningful for the health professional.

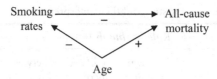

FIGURE 5.2 Depiction of age as a covariate that confounds the association between smoking and mortality (Simpson's paradox).

Adjusting for covariates

Baseline differences between groups can affect the relationship between exposure and outcome. The example of "Simpson's paradox" [3] illustrates how (Figure 5.2).

A study compared women smokers to women non-smokers to observe the effects of smoking on mortality. The study found that fewer smokers (24%) than nonsmokers (31%) had died 20 years after baseline observations were made – smoking appeared to reduce mortality by 7%. How was that explained?

It turns out that the two groups of smokers and non-smokers differed in terms of average age – the non-smoking group was considerably older than the smoking group – older women in the non-smoking group outnumbered their counterparts in the smoking group by 162 to 42. In the study, age is negatively associated with smoking. However, age is positively related to mortality – older folk tend to die at higher rates than younger people. Taken together, It is no surprise that mortality was higher among non-smokers (see Figure 5.2).

Simpson's paradox illustrates how one variable, in this case, age, can interfere with or confound the relationship between exposure and health outcome, in this case, smoking and mortality. Once age – a covariate in the study – was statistically adjusted for, a significant, more plausible relationship appeared – upon the 20-year follow up, the odds of death was found to be 53% higher for smokers than for nonsmokers.

This elementary example illustrates the larger point that groups being compared should be comparable – that is, no important pre-existing group differences interfere or partially account for the relationship between exposure and outcome. The challenge is that group differences are not always known, especially when random sampling or assignment is not employed. Therefore, where possible, studies will measure covariates that might plausibly confound the relationship between health outcomes and exposures. The analysis section will describe operations used to statistically adjust for covariates.

In sum, analytical questions prompt readers to assess how data are analyzed, what statistical operations were used to assess the significance and strength of key relationships between outcomes exposures, or interventions, what covariates were included in the analysis, and importantly, what covariates were missing that might plausibly confound the key relationships being analyzed. What comes of this process of collecting and analyzing quantitative data is reported in the Results section.

The results section – Q6, Q7, and Q8

Q6 How was the sample characterized?

The methods describe the source of the sample population and how the sample was drawn. The major aim is to determine how and to whom the study findings might apply.

Usually, the first table in the Results section characterizes the study sample from which data were collected and analyzed – e.g., the sample size, key attributes, and group differences. The sample forms the basis from which findings about the variable relationships are drawn. Once characterized, readers will evaluate how and to whom study findings might apply, or how well they apply to a specific target population.

Q7 Which relationships were reported to be statistically significant (or not)?

Additional tables, figures, or charts, present information about how outcomes and exposures relate. Relevant tables will show the "p-value" used as a measure of confidence that the relationship found in the sample did (or did not) result from random chance (see Appendix D).

For instance, a study compared cannabis use (an exposure) among participants who were diagnosed with psychosis (cases) to those who were not (controls). Table 5.3 indicates significant differences between cases and controls across several exposures.

Among cases, 65.9% were lifetime cannabis users whereas just 47.3% of those in the control were lifetime users. According to the p-value shown ($p < 0.001$), the likelihood that this difference was due to chance was exceedingly low – less than 1 in 1,000. The null hypothesis would be rejected in favor of the research hypothesis. Thus, the evidence supports an association between diagnosed psychosis and lifetime cannabis use (Box 5.3).

As discussed, p-values indicate the likelihood that the relationship identified in the sample occurred by chance. This p-value does not indicate how strong a relationship is – the size of the effect of one variable on another. Other metrics are used to show how strong a relationship is or its "effect size".

BOX 5.3 ASSOCIATIONS AND CAUSES

The evidence presented in Table 5.3 was generated by a study that used an observational, case-control design (see Chapter 6). While the results support an association between cannabis use and diagnosed psychosis, this evidence is insufficient to infer a *causal* association between the two – i.e., that cannabis use caused the (diagnosed) psychosis. Many other factors might precede or intervene in the relationship to produce the association. One might even argue that people with psychosis seek relief through cannabis, reversing the causal link and inflating the association. To confidently argue for a causal linkage between cannabis use and psychosis one would need corroborating evidence from several studies, along with the identification of mechanisms that account for the connection between the two.

TABLE 5.3 Comparing cases with diagnosed psychosis to controls in terms of lifetime cannabis use [4]

Characteristic	No. (%)		p-value
	Controls (n=1,214)	Cases (n=888)	
Lifetime cannabis use			<0.001
Yes	574 (47.3%)	585 (65.9%)	
No	650 (53.5%)	303 (34.1%)	

Q8 *How strong were the relationships?*

Apart from determining its statistical significance, readers often will seek to identify the strength of the association between a health outcome and exposure – e.g., odds ratios, mean differences, Pearson coefficients. For instance, a study divided participants into four cohorts depending on median steps per day and tracked them over a 20-year period to assess the association between steps per day and all-cause mortality (Table 5.4) [5].

The table shows the adjusted hazard ratio (aHR) for each quartile, for adults 60 years old or older, adjusted by age and sex. Cohort quartile #1 – the lowest 25% in terms of steps per day – serves as the reference against which all-cause mortality of the other quartiles is compared. As shown, the aHR for cohort quartile #2 equals 0.56, indicating 44% lower incidence of mortality compared to quartile #1. An aHR = 0.45 for quartile #3 indicates a 55% lower incidence of mortality compared to quartile #1. Finally, an aHR = 0.35 for quartile #4 indicates a 65% lower incidence of mortality compared to quartile #1.

Thus, not only are each of these differences statistically significant, the reductions in mortality rates also increase with each higher quartile. This steady reduction in mortality corresponding to an increase in steps per day suggests a dose-response relationship between the exposure and health outcome – the higher the dose (e.g., steps per day), the higher the response (decline in all-cause mortality). Although not definitive, a dose-response relationship offers certain evidence favoring a causal connection between exposure and outcome.

BOX 5.4 NON-LINEAR RELATIONSHIPS

To complicate matters, while the evidence supported a dose-response relationship between steps taken and mortality, one can imagine a point where additional steps make little difference in terms of mortality. One might also imagine that the initial increase in steps for the most sedentary would produce the greatest benefits in terms of reducing mortality. This suggests a non-linear relationship where the benefits of additional steps diminish. The data from Table 5.4 suggests a non-linear relationship. The greatest improvement in mortality risk occurred between the lowest and second lowest quartile (44% reduction in risk). Lesser reductions are shown in the third (11% reduction) and fourth (10% reduction) quartiles. This suggests a pattern of diminishing returns for additional steps. Some variation of the law of diminishing returns often characterizes variable relationships.

TABLE 5.4 Steps per day and all-cause mortality, adults ≥ 60 years

Quartile (25%)	Median steps per day	aHR (95% CI) all-cause mortality
#1	2,841	1.00 (referent)
#2	5,217	0.56 (0.34–0.92)
#3	7,116	0.45 (0.37–0.55)
#4	10,501	0.35 (0.28–0.45)

The discussion – Q9 and Q10

Q9 *What were the strengths and limitations of the study?*

Having critically analyzed the results of the study and the methods used to produce them, readers are positioned to identify the strengths and limitations of these findings. The Discussion section highlights the contributions of the findings, along with their limitations. The section connects findings to evidence from similar studies and how they might deepen our understanding of the health topic.

The section will also highlight possible biases in the study, which readers may already have identified. These biases are often associated with sampling and measurement, which skew the findings and limit their applications (Appendix B). These limitations serve as cautions against overgeneralizing and misapplying results.

Q10 *What were the implications of the study for research and practice?*

The concluding paragraphs will identify the implications of the study for future research and practice. These may serve to direct the reader in the application of evidence to practice decisions, but readers will identify their own "takeaway" – a key result or conclusion to be drawn from their critical reading.

Recap

This chapter describes ten questions used to analytically read a quantitative research article. Analytical reading quantitative studies involves asking questions across the four main sections of the research article. The first two – Q1 and Q2 – are often answered during the inspection stage and ask about the article's relevance and study design.

Q3, Q4, and Q5, focus on how data are collected (eligibility criteria for participants and variable measures) and analyzed (statistical procedures). This section is crucial for evaluating the study's validity. Q6, Q7, and Q8 ask about the findings from data collection and analysis process. They inquire about the characteristics of the sample and the nature of the associations (e.g., direction, significance, magnitude) between outcome and exposure.

Finally, Q9 and Q10 ask about the strengths, limitations, and implications of the study. These analytical questions activate the reading process and foster a critical examination of findings from the study, along with their applicability to other groups and settings.

The next chapters discuss the observational and experimental studies and how these ten questions may be used to analyze them.

References

1. van Dellen SA, Wisse B, Mobach MP, Dijkstra A. The effect of a breastfeeding support programme on breastfeeding duration and exclusivity: A quasi-experiment. *BMC Public Health.* 2019;19:993. doi:10.1186/s12889-019-7331-y.
2. Reeves A, McKee M, Mackenbach J, Whitehead M, Stuckler D. Introduction of a national minimum wage reduced depressive symptoms in low-wage workers: A quasi-natural experiment in the UK. *Health Econ.* 2017;26(5):639–655. doi:10.1002/hec.3336.

3. Appleton DR, French JM, Vanderpump MPJ. Ignoring a covariate: An example of Simpson's paradox. *Am Stat*. 1996;50(4):340–341. doi:10.1080/00031305.1996.10473550.
4. di Forti M, Quattrone D, Freeman TP, Tripoli G, Gayer-Anderson C, Quigley H, et al. The contribution of cannabis use to variation in the incidence of psychotic disorder across Europe: The EU-GEI case-control study. *Lancet Psychiatry*. 2019;6(5):427–436. doi:10.1016/S2215-0366(19)30048-3.
5. Paluch AE, Bajpai S, Bassett DR, Carnethon MR, Ekelund U, Evenson KR, et al. Daily steps and all-cause mortality: A meta-analysis of 15 international cohorts. *Lancet Public Health*. 2022;7(3):e219–e228. doi:10.1016/S2468-2667(21)00302-9.

6

UNDERSTANDING OBSERVATIONAL DESIGNS

Overview of observational designs

Observational studies observe and record data on *exposures* and health *outcomes* in their natural settings (not under experimental conditions) to assess how the variables may relate. They do not test the effects of a treatment intervention as they do in experimental studies (Chapter 8). An exposure would include any *risk factor* associated with negative health outcomes or any *protective factor* associated with positive health outcomes. For instance, a diet rich in processed foods tends to increase the risk of obesity or type 2 diabetes, while a nutrient-rich diet tends to protect against osteoarthritis and cardiovascular disease.

There are three main types of observational designs – cross-sectional, case-control, and cohort. Occasionally these designs are combined to create a hybrid study design (see Box 6.1 and Example 7.4). Pigeonholing observational designs can be accomplished by inspecting the article's title and abstract. The title often will indicate which of the three main types of observational design is being used – "cross-sectional", "case-control", or "cohort" designs (Table 6.1).

If the title does not give away the type of observational design, the abstract surely will. Pigeonholing the study as using an observational design should be straightforward.

The quality of the evidence derived from cross-sectional, case-control, and cohort studies differs, however. Understanding the differences in these designs will deepen your

TABLE 6.1 Titles in Observational Designs

Type of design	Title
Cross-sectional	Ecological influences on employees' workplace sedentary behavior: a cross-sectional study [1]
Case-control	The contribution of cannabis use to variation in the incidence of psychotic disorder across Europe (EU-GEI): a multicentre case-control study [2]
Cohort	A 2-year prospective cohort study of overuse running injuries [3]

DOI: 10.4324/9781003595663-8

understanding of the results they yield and, consequently, will help target your reading toward studies that are more suitable to your reading purpose. Thus, a clear understanding of the results of these studies presupposes understanding how these designs differ. Each design is discussed below.

BOX 6.1 HYBRID DESIGNS

There are occasions where researchers combine different research designs. These hybrid designs are also called "blended", "mixed", or "integrated" designs. Quantitative and qualitative designs serve to complement each other in *mixed-methods* designs (see Example 9.2). Hybrid studies may merge case-control and cohort designs in a single study (see Example 7.4).

Understanding cross-sectional designs

Cross-sectional design is the most basic of observational designs – data is collected at one time and then they are analyzed. Figure 6.1 depicts a cross-sectional design.

Cross-sectional studies provide a description of the population at a particular point in time – a snapshot, not a video. Since data are collected once, cross-sectional studies, as a rule, take less time to conduct than other designs.

Cross-sectional designs often use online questionnaires to collect survey data for analysis. For instance, a one-time survey might find that, on average, those who spend more time on social media, on average, also report higher levels of anxiety – social media use and anxiety increase or decline together. Since both variables are assessed at the same time, we cannot say that change in social media use *causes* change in anxiety levels. Neither can we say that that change in anxiety levels *causes* people to turn to social media. Perhaps the two variables are mutually reinforcing or perhaps another, third variable causes both to change at the same time. Either way, a cross-sectional study may show variables to be associated, but not *causally* related. Correlation is a necessary but insufficient condition to infer causality.

Many cross-sectional studies are routinely conducted to collect and update data on certain topics. These studies may be ongoing governmental surveys – e.g., the Health Survey for England (HSE), the Canadian Community Health Survey (CCHS), the Australian Health Survey (AHS), and the National Health Interview Survey (NHIS). For instance, the CDC's National Health and Nutrition Examination Survey (NHANES) routinely collects cross-sectional data on variables regarding diet and health behaviors

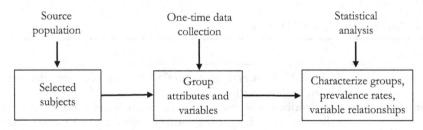

FIGURE 6.1 The structure of the cross-sectional design.

(see Box 6.2). Data from these surveys may serve as secondary data that researchers can draw from for their own analysis (see Box 3.3). Researchers can curate and analyze already-collected, secondary data. For instance, a study of the use of dietary supplements drew from NHANES data and reported a 50% increase in the use of dietary supplements and micronutrient products among US adults [4]. Three studies used to illustrate different observational designs rely on the analysis of secondary data (Chapter 7).

BOX 6.2 THE NHANES SURVEY

The National Health and Nutrition Examination Survey (NHANES) is an ongoing survey designed to assess the health and nutrition status of *all* non-institutionalized adults and children in the US. This involves complex multistage random (probability) sampling to assure that the sample represents the larger study population. NHANES researchers randomly select primary sampling units – geographic regions – and randomly selected subareas and sub-subareas within these regions. This eventually leads to a randomly chosen household and individual within the household. In 2015–2016, 15,327 individuals were selected to represent the nation's 300 million-plus population (.005%). Certain subgroups are over-sampled to ensure adequate representation.

Strengths and limitations of cross-sectional studies

Compared to other designs, cross-sectional designs are less expensive to complete, and the results are more readily available. Cross-sectional studies provide a snapshot of the landscape of disease, risks, health, and illness that can be useful for planning and monitoring. They can help us gauge the *burden of disease* and the importance of addressing this burden (see Box 6.3). They may also show how multiple variables interact, identifying numerous direct and indirect associations. Although cross-sectional studies cannot establish a causal relationship, they serve to support causal connections found in other studies and may also serve as a starting point for exploring exposure-outcome relationships using other designs.

Cross-sectional designs offer a practical way to survey the attitudes, attributes, and behaviors of large populations. By selecting a random sample from a larger population, findings may be generalized to this larger population. On the other hand, readers should remain cautious about possible selection biases surveys where only a small percentage of people respond. A 10% response rate risks producing results that are skewed toward, for instance, more eager, more literate, and more connected respondents who have a keen interest in the topic, while other groups and perspectives are under-represented.

Cross-sectional studies often use questionnaires that gather certain information indirectly, requiring respondents to self-report events, attitudes, and behaviors. This introduces potential for various self-report biases (Appendix B). For instance, respondents may incorrectly recall events or behaviors (recall bias) or respond in socially acceptable ways may skew the data toward what is perceived as accepted or desirable rather than what is true (social desirability bias).

BOX 6.3 BURDEN OF DISEASE

The burden of disease encompasses the evaluation of the financial and human costs of morbidity and mortality. The evaluation informs the rationale regarding research questions and objectives, as well as decisions concerning the development of practice guidelines (Chapter 14). Importantly, the evaluation will inform decisions concerning the allocation of resources toward research and funding aimed to reduce these burdens.

Understanding case-control designs

Case-control designs begin by identifying "cases" where a health outcome is present along with a set of (matched) "controls" where the outcome is absent. Once cases (where the outcome is present) and controls (where it is not) are identified, the two groups are compared by looking backward at past exposures. The expectation usually is that cases will report significantly more or significantly fewer exposures than controls, suggesting that exposure is associated with a health outcome. Figure 6.2 depicts the structure of the case-control design.

It is important that cases and controls are as similar as possible in other ways. Ideally, cases and controls are drawn from the same population. Where feasible, once cases have been identified, controls may be matched with cases according to certain characteristics – e.g., gender, age, and education. Matching cases with controls across several variables enhances the comparability of the two groups in terms of exposure (see Box 6.4).

For instance, to assess the relationship between skin melanoma and indoor tanning, a study identified patients diagnosed with skin melanoma and randomly selected age-matched and gender-matched controls taken from state driver's license lists [5]. Cases and controls were then compared in terms of prior exposures to indoor tanning. You might expect that cases would report more exposure to indoor tanning than controls, a hypothesis that, in this study, was supported.

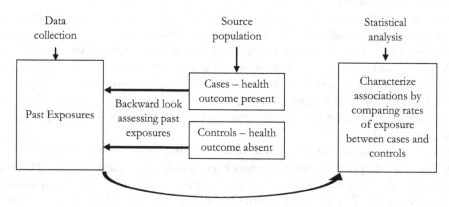

FIGURE 6.2 The structure of the case-control design.

BOX 6.4 MATCHED CONTROLS

Studies will use a matching process to improve the balance between individuals and groups where the health outcome is present or absent. Where possible, the matching process will randomly select participants in the control group from a larger population. The methodological aim is to make groups being compared equivalent in terms of all relevant variables except for the exposure. Matching often occurs along age and gender lines, but several more variables may be included in the matching process.

Skin melanomas are comparatively rare and can take decades to develop. By starting with existing cases, the study eliminates the need to wait for these rare, slowly progressing health conditions to emerge. Case-control designs can also rapidly identify risks of exposure to fast-developing outbreaks of infectious disease or illness. For instance, a case-control study collected data early on in the COVID-19 pandemic (July 2020) to compare cases that tested positive for SARS-CoV-2 to controls that tested negative in terms of close-contact exposures (e.g., restaurants, gyms, salons, and public transportation) during 14 days prior to the positive test [6]. Compared to controls, cases were twice as likely to report having dined in a restaurant during the past 2 weeks. On the other hand, exposure to shopping, home gatherings, and public transport was not shown to relate to positive COVID-19 testing. Although not definitive, the case-control study offered early clues and warnings about the kind of contact the population should or should not avoid (see Example 7.2).

Strengths and limitations of case-control studies

Unlike cross-sectional studies, case-control designs add an important time dimension to the study and can offer initial evidence that an exposure affects an outcome. Once cases and controls are identified, the researcher can explore multiple exposures and examine their association with the health outcome. The design is useful for studying rare outcomes that take time to develop. It also enables a rapid assessment of possible risks associated with sudden outbreaks of a disease or condition.

Case-control designs often rely on research subjects to recall past exposures, and are, therefore, susceptible to recall bias (Appendix B). Inaccurate memories often cloud the resulting data, and the more distant the data to be recalled, the cloudier the memories become. Also, certain exposures may be more salient and memorable for affected cases than unaffected controls, possibly skewing the comparisons. This can introduce recall bias where cases may report exposures more frequently and accurately than controls. For instance, individuals with melanoma (cases) may be more likely to recall and report exposures to indoor tanning than controls. Likewise, individuals with COVID-19 (cases) are more inclined to recall and report prior exposures (e.g., restaurant dining) than controls.

To avoid biases associated with measures that are based on self-report, case-control studies often rely on existing secondary data collected over time to access data about exposures. For instance, a *hybrid study* used publicly available records from 1980 to

2017 to compare NBA players who experienced ACL injury (cases) to players who did not (controls) regarding prior exposures (Example 7.4) [7]. Reliance on secondary data may have its own biases, however, depending on the reliability and validity with which the data were initially collected.

Understanding cohort study designs

Whereas case-control designs compare outcomes with respect to prior exposures, cohort studies compare exposures with respect to future outcomes. This temporal sequence – from exposure to health outcome – aligns with the sequence required for making a causal inference about the association between exposure and outcome. Figure 6.3 depicts the structure of cohort designs.

For instance, using secondary data on birth and death records from Ontario's vital statistics, a cohort study tracked over 3 million children, adolescents, and young adults (age 1–24) born from 1990 to 2016 in five income groups (quintiles) to assess the risk of death (outcome) based on mother's income [8].

The highest income quintile (top 20%) was used as the referent against which other quintiles were compared. The hazard ratio (HR) estimates shown in Table 6.2 were adjusted for attributes of the child (e.g., sex and congenital anomalies) and the birth mother (e.g., world region of origin and age).

The results show that the HR for mortality increased as income decreased. For instance, the adjusted HR for Q1, the lowest quintile, compared to Q5, the highest quintile, is 1.39, with a 95% CI from 1.29 to 1.51. Translated, the incidence of death was, on

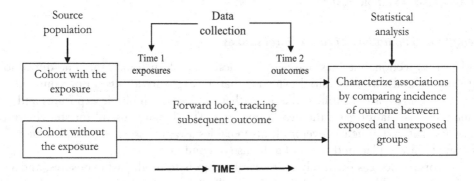

FIGURE 6.3 The structure of the cohort design.

TABLE 6.2 Incidence of death among persons 1–24 years of age, by income quintile (1990–2016)

Residential income quintile	Adjusted HR (95% CI)
Highest 20% – Q5	1.00 (referent)
Q4	1.02 (0.94–1.10)
Q3	1.05 (0.97–1.14)
Q2	1.12 (1.03–1.21)
Lowest 20% – Q1	1.39 (1.29–1.51)

average, 39% higher among children born in the lowest income quintile compared to the highest quintile. Other quintiles show a smaller difference from Q5.

As with other observational designs, *retrospective* cohort designs are often based on previously collected secondary data. In comparison, *prospective* cohort designs collect original data from cohorts and track outcomes into the future (see Box 6.5).

BOX 6.5   RETROSPECTIVE AND PROSPECTIVE COHORT STUDIES

Retrospective cohort studies use secondary data to assess the association between exposures and outcomes. In contrast, prospective cohort studies follow subjects forward in time, from exposure to outcomes. The famous Framingham Heart Study has collected primary data – e.g., demographic, medical, environmental, psychological, and behavioral – from its original cohort in 1948, and followed up with second (1971) and third (2002) generation cohorts. This study has taught and continues to teach us much of what we know about risk and protective factors associated with heart health [9].

Strengths and Limitations of Cohort Studies

The cohort design offers advantages over cross-sectional and case-control observational designs. Cross-sectional designs offer a one-time snapshot and, therefore, cannot indicate the direction of the relationship (e.g., from exposure to outcome). Case-control studies offer a backward look from outcome to exposure, where the "effect" (outcome) is examined to determine a preceding "cause" (exposure). In contrast, cohort studies collect data from exposure to outcome – at baseline, where the entire study population is free of the outcome and can only experience it later (see Figure 6.4). The temporal sequence aligns with the direction of cause and effect. Cohort designs allow us to determine how many new cases (incidents) arise over time and offer a clearer determination of the risk or hazard associated with a given exposure.

Case-control and cohort designs differ in another way – case-control designs can examine multiple exposures for a single outcome, whereas cohort designs can track several outcomes associated with a single exposure. A case-control study might look back on the prior community exposures that might relate to positive tests for COVID-19. In contrast, a cohort study would look forward to tracking the effects of COVID-19 on brain fog, respiratory ailments, cardiovascular ailments, and death.

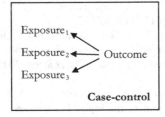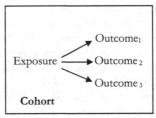

FIGURE 6.4   Case-control designs – many exposures per outcome; Cohort designs – many outcomes per exposure.

One drawback of cohort designs is their costs – following a cohort over time is often expensive and impractical, particularly when tracking outcomes over long periods of time. Cohort designs often use secondary data to study certain outcomes, though the data may not be available or accessible.

Cohort studies also confront the problem of attrition. Over time, participants drop out or otherwise are "lost to follow up". Not only does this reduce your pool of subjects, but the loss of cases may not be random. For instance, attrition may occur when data are missing from a record, which effectively removes the case from the analysis. The study of the incidence of death by income quintile removed over 17 thousand cases due to missing data on income. An aHR = 1.58 was found for these cases. While we might assume that this higher HR would suggest that these missing values were from low or very low-income groups, but we cannot know this for sure.

Recap

This chapter outlined the fundamental concepts and methodologies associated with observational research designs. It suggested that observational designs are especially useful for determining risk or protective factors associated with health outcomes as observed in natural settings. In this regard, observational designs improve the ability to predict health outcomes based on exposures and are well-suited for "upstream" approaches designed to promote health and prevent illness. Observational designs greatly contribute to our understanding and knowledge of public health and epidemiology.

The Chapter also described the three main types of observational designs– cross-sectional, case-control, and cohort study designs. Each of the designs uniquely characterizes the association between exposures and health outcomes. The cross-sectional design offers a snapshot of a population's health at a single point in time to initially characterize the relationship between variables. Case-control designs identify individuals with and without a health outcome (cases and controls) and look backward to observe various associations with various exposures. Third, cohort designs follow groups with different exposures (i.e., cohorts) over time to observe their relationships with health outcomes.

Finally, the Chapter discusses the strengths and limitations of each design. It maintains that understanding these strengths and limitations fosters a clearer and more discerning perspective regarding the implications of the findings for research and practice.

References

1. Wilkerson AH, Usdan SL, Knowlden AP, Leeper JL, Birch DA, Hibberd EE. Ecological influences on employees' workplace sedentary behavior: A cross-sectional study. *Am J Health Promot*. 2018;32(8):1688–1696. doi:10.1177/0890117118767717.
2. di Forti M, Quattrone D, Freeman TP, Tripoli G, Gayer-Anderson C, Quigley H, et al. The contribution of cannabis use to variation in the incidence of psychotic disorder across Europe (EU-GEI): A multicentre case-control study. *Lancet Psychiatry*. 2019;6(5):427–436. doi:10.1016/S2215-0366(19)30048-3.
3. Messier SP, Martin DF, Mihalko SL, Ip E, Devita P, Cannon DW, et al. A 2-year prospective cohort study of overuse running injuries: The Runners and Injury Longitudinal Study (TRAILS). *Am J Sports Med*. 2018;46(9):2211–2221. doi:10.1177/0363546518773755.

4. Cowan AE, Tooze JA, Gahche JJ, Eicher-Miller HA, Guenther PM, Dwyer JT, et al. Trends in overall and micronutrient-containing dietary supplement use in US adults and children, NHANES 2007–2018. *J Nutr*. 2022;152(12):2789–2801. doi:10.1093/jn/nxac168.
5. Lazovich D, Vogel RI, Berwick M, Weinstock MA, Anderson KE, Warshaw EM. Indoor tanning and risk of melanoma: A case-control study in a highly exposed population. *Cancer Epidemiol Biomarkers Prev*. 2010;19(6):1557–1568. doi:10.1158/1055-9965.EPI-09-1249.
6. Fisher KA, Tenforde MW, Feldstein LR, Lindsell CJ, Shapiro NI, Files DC, et al. Community and close contact exposures associated with COVID-19 among symptomatic adults ≥18 years in 11 outpatient health care facilities — United States, July 2020. *MMWR Morb Mortal Wkly Rep*. 2020;69(36):1258–1264. doi:10.15585/mmwr.mm6936a5.
7. Schultz BJ, Thomas KA, Cinque M, Harris JD, Maloney WJ, Abrams GD. Tendency of driving to the basket is associated with increased risk of anterior cruciate ligament tears in National Basketball Association players: A cohort study. *Orthop J Sports Med*. 2021;9(11). doi:10.1177/23259671211052953.
8. Ray JG, Guttmann A, Silveira J, Park AL. Mortality in a cohort of 3.1 million children, adolescents, and young adults. *J Epidemiol Community Health*. 2020;74(3):260–268. doi:10.1136/jech-2019-213365.
9. Tsao CW, Vasan RS. Cohort profile: The Framingham Heart Study (FHS): Overview of milestones in cardiovascular epidemiology. *Int J Epidemiol*. 2015;44(6):1800–1813. doi:10.1093/ije/dyv337.

7

ANALYTICALLY READING OBSERVATIONAL STUDIES

Chapter 6 provided an overview of three observational designs. Chapter 5 identified ten (10) questions to ask of primary studies that take a quantitative approach. This chapter illustrates the process of analytically reading peer-reviewed studies that use observational designs – cross-sectional, case-control, and cohort. A fourth example illustrates the critical examination of a study that uses a case-control/cohort hybrid design.

Example 7.1 Analytically reading a cross-sectional study

Title: "Health behaviors of American pregnant women: a cross-sectional analysis of NHANES 2007–2014" [1].

This example illustrates the use of secondary data – previously collected data that is available to others to curate and analyze. In this study, data was drawn from the CDC's National Health and Nutrition Examination Survey (NHANES). The survey has been ongoing since 1999, but earlier cycles data back to the early 1960s.

The study curates NHANES data collected from 2007 to 2014. Since the NHANES program randomly selects a new sample each year, the study cannot track change in individuals or cohorts over time.

Rather, these were data from single observations (an interview or physical examination) of different individuals (in this case, pregnant women) recorded during that timeframe. Thus, the study uses cross-sectional data and illustrates a cross-sectional design.

Inspectional reading

Readers will already have answered the first two analytical questions based on the title, abstract, and introduction.

DOI: 10.4324/9781003595663-9

Q1 Is the study relevant (with respect to your current aims)? and

Q2 What study design was used?

By inspecting the title, you can tell what the study is about – i.e., health behaviors of American pregnant women. You can tell the design used was cross-sectional – "a cross-sectional analysis of…". Survey data comes from NHANES (2007–2014).

The Introduction argues the importance of healthy behaviors during pregnancy, citing studies that support the argument. In then identifies deficiencies in what we know about the health behaviors of pregnant women to set up the principal objective of the study: "to examine engagement in five recommended health behaviors".

Seeking to go beyond the summary description provided in the abstract, readers will actively examine the full text of the study to obtain answers to the other analytic questions to help inform them and to deepen their understanding of the strengths, limits, and implications of the study.

Reading the methods

Q3 What inclusion/exclusion criteria did the study use to select the sample?

The study population consists of pregnant women in the US who participated in the NHANES study from 2007 to 2014. NHANES survey data comes from both interviews and physical examination. The article briefly describes the data as cross-sectional, aiming to represent all non-institutionalized residents in the US. The article refers interested readers to a CDC website for a detailed description of the methods, including the multi-stage, random sampling process used to generate the study sample.

In assessing the inclusion/ exclusion criteria, readers seek to understand how results from the study population might be relevant to the population of their interest. In this example, the study used random sampling to represent pregnant women in the United States. While the random sample might well represent behaviors of pregnant women in the US, it poorly reflects behaviors of pregnant women elsewhere – say, Canada, Mexico, the UK, Italy, India, or China. Thus, the evidence from this descriptive study might be valuable for health professionals in the US, but less so for health professionals elsewhere.

Finally, it is worth considering when the article was published or, specifically, when data was collected. In this example, data was collected over 10 years ago. Readers might then wonder whether recommended health behaviors might have changed during this time, and how or why the health behaviors of American pregnant women might have changed or evolved since then.

Q4 How valid and reliable were the variable measures?

Following a description of the data source (NHANES) and the study population (pregnant women in the US), the article describes the ways in which the study measures demographic variables, pregnancy status (interview and physical examination), and each of five recommended health behaviors – fruit and vegetable consumption, prenatal multivitamin use, physical activity, sleep duration, and smoking status.

NHANES measured health behaviors through participants' self-reports. For instance, consumption of fruit and vegetables was gauged by taking the average of two 24-hour dietary recalls. Physical activity was measured based on self-reports of frequency, duration, and exertion level for work and leisure activities. The measures are subject to recall and social desirability biases that serve as an added source of variation in the data (Appendix B). Notwithstanding this limitation, the use of these measures is supported by other studies referenced in the article.

Q5 *How were the data analyzed?*

This article reports how the study transformed health behavior data into binary data (dichotomies) – whether respondents did or did not adhere to the behavioral recommendations. The study would present descriptive results regarding the five behavior recommendations – e.g., estimates of frequency, cumulative number of recommended behaviors.

Dichotomizing variables into two categories (e.g., respondents did or did not adhere to behavior recommendations) also enables the use of ratios to describe and present the results. For instance, the study used an odds ratio (OR) to compare the odds of engaging in a behavior between groups – e.g., respondents with some college education versus respondents with no college education.

Finally, the analysis subsection describes the use of multivariate logistic regression models to estimate frequency of adherence to a behavior while adjusting for other covariates – age, race/ethnicity, income, education, marital status.

Reading the results

Q6 *How was the sample characterized?*

The methods section defines how the sample is selected and from what source population. The resulting sample is typically characterized in the first table in the Results section. In this article, the table and corresponding text report the frequency and number of respondents by categories of age, ethnicity, income, education, and marital status. The table shows the sample size ($n = 248$) and variation in the data across groups – e.g., 65% had at least some college, 77% were married or living with a partner, and 20% reported household incomes less than $20,000. This provides additional context for understanding how the data might apply to the groups or individuals the reader is targeting.

Q7 *Which relationships were reported to be statistically significant (or not)?*

The study identified the portion with which pregnant women met each health behavior guideline – adequate fruit/vegetable consumption (35%), prenatal vitamins (62%), physical activity (73%), adequate sleep (72%), and non-smoking (87%). For all recommended behaviors, the difference between those who did or did not adhere was statistically significant ($p \leq 0.001$). In other words, it was highly unlikely that this difference was due to chance.

TABLE 7.1 Adherence to recommended health behaviors by age and race/ethnicity of pregnant women

Characteristic	Adherence		Multivariate model for adherence	
	Yes	No	OR (95% CI)	p-value
Age (years)	29.42	28.37	1.03 (0.97–1.09)	0.40
Race/ethnicity				
Non-Hispanic White	37.82	56.16	1.00 (referent)	
Non-Hispanic Black	14.72	18.93	1.39 (0.51–3.80)	0.52
Hispanic	26.42	16.72	3.69 (1.47–9.25)	0.01
Other	21.02	8.19	3.36 (1.17–9.66)	0.03

Adapted from "Characteristics of pregnant women ($N = 248$)". Data from [1].

The study also compared adherence to guidelines regarding fruit and vegetable consumption using adjusted ORs to indicate differences. Table 7.1 (modified from the original) compares adherence to fruit and vegetable guidelines by age and race/ethnicity.

The rightmost column identifies group differences that are statistically significant – where the p-value is less than 0.05. The Table shows a difference with respect to the average age of adherents and non-adherents to the fruit and vegetable recommendation. Adherents were only slightly older on average – 29.42 years to 28.37 years – but the difference is not large enough to rule out chance as a plausible explanation for the (insignificant) difference ($p = 0.40$).

In contrast, the p-value for adherence for Hispanic women, and for women classified as "Other" was low – $p = 0.01$ and $p = 0.03$. That is, the observed difference between Non-Hispanic White women (the referent) and Hispanic women and women classified with respect to adherence was unlikely due to chance. Finally, adherence to recommendation did not differ significantly for Non-Hispanic White and Non-Hispanic Black women – $p = 0.52$).

Q8 How strong were the relationships?

Based on the p-values presented in column 5, we learned that the observed difference between pregnant Hispanic and Non-Hispanic White women was unlikely due to chance. While this finding suggests that there is a real difference between the groups, it does not indicate how substantial this difference is.

The fourth column in Table 7.1 uses adjusted odds ratios (ORs) to suggest the size of this difference between the groups with respect to the consumption of fruit and vegetables. Recall that an OR compares odds of an event occurring in one group compared to another group. For this example, this would compare the odds of adherence among pregnant Hispanic women to the odds among pregnant non-Hispanic White women, adjusted for covariates (e.g., marital status, income, education, and age). The observed odds of adherence – aOR = 3.69 – were 3.69 times higher for pregnant Hispanic women compared to pregnant non-Hispanic White women.

Of course, there is substantial variation among pregnant women in both groups, and this is reflected in the wide confidence intervals (CIs) presented along with the aOR – (95%

CI = 1.47, 9.25). Thus, while the observed differences between groups were substantial and statistically significant there is considerable variation within these groups. Numerous other factors affect behavior and may account for the variation surrounding the point-estimate. No doubt various ecological, economic, social, and cultural factors combine to affect diet and fruit and vegetable consumption. Additional studies would be needed to refine our knowledge of the factors that affect health behaviors.

Reading the discussion

Q9 *What were the strengths and limitations of the study?*

This study aimed to identify the frequency of certain health behaviors among pregnant women in the US. It did not attempt to identify factors that encourage or discourage these behaviors among women. It primarily described the frequency of certain behaviors rather than explained them. The description, however, is useful for identifying the magnitude of the health issue and for targeting efforts to encourage healthy behaviors toward groups less likely to engage in recommended behaviors.

The article described the cross-sectional design as a primary weakness. As a snapshot of health behaviors of pregnant women, the study is unable to assess how these behaviors may change during the course of the pregnancy. Diet and activity levels might vary from one trimester to the next during a pregnancy, and this could not be accounted for in the study.

Finally, the study relied largely on self-reported measures of health behaviors. For instance, data for fruit and vegetable intake relied on 24-hour dietary recall. Since direct observation of diet is rare, reliance on such self-reported measures is as common. Although the 24-hour recall may offer the best, most feasible way to assess dietary intake, inaccurate memory, and social desirability bias adds variation in reporting fruit and vegetable intake. Self-reports of other behaviors pose similar risks and contribute to unexplained variation in the findings.

Q10 *What were the implications of this study for research and practice?*

The Discussion concludes that, despite these limitations, the study updates the reader on the frequency of various health behaviors among pregnant women. The study found that a small portion of pregnant women followed the recommendations for fruit and vegetable intake, and just half reported taking prenatal multivitamins in the last 30 days. On the plus side, these health behaviors are modifiable, so the deficiency can be addressed.

Readers take away a description of the frequency with which pregnant women in the US adhere to behavioral recommendations and determine that overall adherence was moderate at best. Public health professionals, dieticians, and other professionals might offer advice or target programs to certain groups to foster healthier behaviors during pregnancy.

Example 7.2   Analytically reading a case-control study

Title: "Community and Close Contact Exposures Associated with COVID-19 Among Symptomatic Adults ≥ 18 Years in 11 Outpatient Health Care Facilities – United States, July 2020" [2].

A second example is a case-control study conducted by the US Centers for Disease Control (CDC) about close-contact exposures that might contribute to the spread of SARS-Cov-2 (COVID-19). By mid-2020, the virus had already spread rapidly, resulting in a significant increase in morbidity and mortality rates. As a novel virus, we had little understanding of how it was transmitted. The case-control design enabled swift collection, analysis, and dissemination of data, which, while imperfect, offered early evidence to inform responses to the ongoing pandemic.

The study was published in the CDC's Morbidity and Mortality Weekly Report (MMWR). The CDC's MMWR is part of the substantial "gray" literature (see Box 3.2). The MMWR undergoes internal, CDC review by qualified professionals, but not the impartial external review that characterizes peer-reviewed articles. The large team of investigators reported no financial or non-financial conflicts of interest (see Box 7.1). As the title suggests, the study investigated "community and contact exposures" associated with the pandemic's spread.

BOX 7.1   CONFLICTS OF INTEREST

A conflict of interest arises when an individual's multiple interests are in opposition. This is often seen in research when a scientist maintains a professional duty to conduct objective research yet holds a personal or financial interest in obtaining favorable results. While scientists strive to maintain objectivity, the financial support from the funder can create a conflict, possibly influencing the study's outcomes to avoid jeopardizing future funding. Consequently, conflicts of interest are recognized as potential sources of bias. To bolster the integrity and transparency of the research, it is essential that authors disclose any conflicts of interest.

Inspectional reading

The study's relevance during the early phase of the pandemic is self-evident – public health officials and the public at large needed to know how close contacts might contribute to the spread of the novel COVID-19 virus. The specific observational design used is evident in the first paragraph:

> To assess community and close contact exposures associated with COVID-19, exposures reported by case-patients (154) were compared with exposures reported by control-participants (160) [2].

Reading the methods

Q3 *What inclusion/exclusion criteria did the study use to select the sample?*

The article described how cases and controls were identified. Cases and controls came from 11 healthcare sites in the US. Case-patients were symptomatic adults confirmed to have SARS-CoV-2 infection from among the sites. Control-participants were symptomatic adults from the same facilities who tested negative. For each case-patient, two adult control-patients were selected, matched by age, sex, and study location. (Later we learn that not all controls were eligible or completed the interview process, so an unmatched analysis was performed.)

Q4 *How valid and reliable were the variable measures?*

The outcome variable was defined by the SARS-CoV-2 test result – i.e., case-patients who tested positive and control-patients who tested negative. Positive cases were confirmed using laboratory testing.

Data on exposures were collected through structured interviews and relied on self-reports. Cases and controls were asked about their community and close-contact exposures (defined as within 6 feet for 15 minutes or more) during the 14 days prior to the onset of disease. They were also asked about mask-wearing behaviors.

Reliance on self-reports introduces the risk of bias and contributes to variation in the data. Recalling past events can be challenging and participants vary in their ability to do so accurately. Moreover, recall might be sharper for positive cases, for whom previous contacts would be particularly memorable. In contrast, negative cases would be more likely to forget about or overlook past exposures, since these contacts did not lead to significant negative outcomes. This could lead to an over-reporting of close-contact exposures among positive cases compared to negative controls.

Q5 *How were the data analyzed?*

A logistical regression analysis would be used to compute an OR comparing cases and controls in terms of reported exposures. The ORs were adjusted for age, sex, race/ethnicity, and chronic conditions. Logistic regression analysis is frequently used to produce adjusted ORs that compare cases and controls in terms of exposures, while controlling for potential confounding variables.

Reading the results

Q6 *How was the sample characterized?*

The text and table described the sample size – $n = 154$ for cases, $n = 160$ for controls – and compared the groups in terms of age, sex, race/ethnicity, education, medical conditions, and exposures. The table compared cases and controls indicate no statistically significant differences in terms of age ($p = 0.18$) or sex ($p = 0.51$). Significant differences were shown for race/ethnicity ($p < 0.01$) and education ($p < 0.01$) – controls were significantly more likely to be White, non-Hispanic, and to have a college degree or higher.

TABLE 7.2 Community and contact exposures among positive and negative Covid-19 cases

Community exposure	Cases	Controls	p-value
Shopping	131 (85.6)	141 (88.1)	0.51
Home, ≤10 persons	79 (51.3)	84 (52.5)	0.83
Restaurant	63 (40.9)	44 (27.7)	0.01
Office setting	37 (24.0)	47 (29.6)	0.27
Salon	24 (15.6)	28 (17.6)	0.63
Home > 10 persons	21 (13.6)	24 (15.0)	0.73
Gym	12 (7.8)	10 (6.3)	0.60
Public transportation	8 (5.2)	10 (6.3)	0.68
Bar/coffee shop	13 (8.5)	8 (5.0)	0.22
Church/religious gathering	12 (7.8)	8 (5.0)	0.32

Adapted from "Community and Close Contact Exposures Associated with COVID-19 among Symptomatic Adults ≥18 Years in 11 Outpatient Health Care Facilities United States, July 2020". Data from [2].

Q7 Which relationships were statistically significant (or not)?

Table 7.2 shows observed differences between cases and controls in community exposures over the 14 days prior to illness.

Differences between cases and controls in terms of all but one exposure were not statistically significant – chance could not be ruled out as a plausible explanation for the difference. Exposure to restaurant dining was the lone exception – $p = 0.01$. In sum, the findings supported an association between restaurant dining and testing positive for COVID-19 but did not support an association for the other nine exposures examined.

Q8 How strong were the relationships?

Statistical significance does not signify the strength of the relationship – e.g., how much *more likely* is it that cases will report restaurant dining than controls? This study used adjusted odds ratios (aORs) to estimate the strength of the associations (adjusted for age, race/ethnicity, sex, and chronic conditions). The article reported that:

…case-patients were more likely to have reported dining at a restaurant (aOR = 2.4, 95% CI = 1.5–3.8) in the 2 weeks before illness onset than were control-participants.

Thus, the odds of having dined in a restaurant prior to testing positive for COVID-19 was, on average, 2.4 times greater for cases compared to controls (aOR = 2.4). This point-estimate is surrounded by 95% CIs, suggesting that the true population parameter likely lies somewhere between 1.5 and 3.8 (see Box 7.2).

For some exposures the differences might be considered sizeable – e.g., the odds of having been exposed to a bar/coffee shop were over 2.5 times greater for cases compared to controls. However, the absolute number of exposures was too small to discount random chance as an explanation.

BOX 7.2 95% CIS AND STATISTICAL SIGNIFICANCE

Confidence intervals are typically presented alongside ratios (ORs, RRs, and HRs) to provide a range in the estimate of the true population parameter. Ratios equal to 1.0 indicate that there is no difference between the groups (Appendix F). From the CIs, one can identify if a ratio is statistically significant. The rule is simple: If 1.0 falls within the upper and lower limit of the CI, then the result is not statistically significant – i.e., it is plausible that differences were due to chance. In contrast, if the 95% CI does not encompass 1.0, then the association is statistically significant – it is implausible (less than 5% likelihood) that the difference between groups with respect to exposure or outcome is due to chance.

Reading the discussion

Q9 What were the strengths and limitations of the study?

One strength was that the case-control design allowed for comparatively rapid turnaround with respect to potential risks of exposure. Given the gravity of the COVID-19 outbreak, this rapid turnaround was important for informing the public about these risks. The study provides early evidence of the risk of various exposures on COVID-19.

As a case-control design, however, data on community exposures were collected retrospectively. A causal linkage between restaurant dining and positive tests for COVID-19 could not be made. Further, researchers used self-reports to identify exposures, adding to the risk of bias associated with self-reported measures. This contributes to variation in the findings. The interviews did not distinguish between indoor and outdoor dining, a limitation that later studies would need to address. Finally, SARS-CoV-2 tests were subject to false negatives and positives that might result in misclassifying cases and controls.

Q10 What were the implications of the study for research and practice?

Restaurants, bars, and coffee shops appear to be at higher risk, perhaps due to air circulation, the inability to mask while eating or drinking, and challenges with physical distancing. This knowledge helped inform policies and practices relative to the pandemic.

Example 7.3 Analytically reading a cohort study

Title: "Association of cardiorespiratory fitness with long-term mortality among adults undergoing exercise treadmill testing" [3].

This example illustrates a (retrospective) cohort study that uses secondary data from medical records to divide patients into five cohorts based on performance on a test of cardiorespiratory fitness. These cohorts were then followed over time to assess, as the title reads, the long-term mortality.

Inspectional reading

Readers will already have answered the first two analytical questions based on the title, abstract, and introduction. The title specifies the health outcome – all-cause mortality – and exposure – cardiorespiratory fitness (CRF). The abstract indicates that the study uses a cohort design to explore the relationship between the two. The Introduction described deficiencies in measures other studies had used to assess the relationship between CRF and mortality. Specifically, some studies suggested that the beneficial effects would level off or decline for the highest CRF groups. Therefore, a major study objective was to assess the association between CRF and mortality in a large study population which included elite CRF performers.

Reading the methods

Q3 *What inclusion/exclusion criteria did the study use to select the sample?*

The study curated data from medical records on adult patients who underwent treadmill testing between January 1991 and 2014. The data provides the opportunity to track a large number of patients forward in time over a maximum of 24 years.

The hospital from which records were drawn was located in the midwestern US. While adult US Midwesterners will differ in many ways from people living elsewhere, it is less clear how the biological mechanisms that would account for the relationship between CRF and mortality would operate differently in other populations. If not, findings from this study population might apply more generally than, say, findings from the NHANES study on health behaviors of pregnant women.

Q4 *How valid and reliable were the variable measures?*

The medical record supplied the patient's demographic information, anthropometric data (e.g., weight, height, and BMI), medications, and comorbidities. These measures involved extracting information recorded in medical records and social security files. The health outcome – all-cause mortality – was based on the Social Security Death Index and on information about the patient's death recorded in the medical record.

Data on the exposure – cardiorespiratory fitness (CRF) – was based on the patient's performance on exercise treadmill test (ETT) and quantified as peak estimated metabolic equivalents (METs). The treadmill test was administered using a standard testing protocol and monitored by the local exercise physiologists. This enhanced the consistency of measures. Based on CRF test performance, five cohorts were constructed – low, below average, above average, high, and elite categories. Once cohorts were established, subjects in each category were monitored until death or the conclusion of the study. Thus, the study could compare mortality rates for each of the five CRF cohorts.

Q5 *How were the data analyzed?*

The cohort study examines records over 24 years, with subjects entering and dying throughout. To assess the influence of CRF on mortality, therefore, the analysis must not only consider *that* a subject died, but *when* they died relative to when they entered the study. Results from this survival analysis are also presented in terms of hazard ratios (HRs) in the Results section (see Appendix F).

Baseline differences among these groups were adjusted for by the inclusion of covariates in a multivariate regression model. These covariates were: age, sex, BMI, various comorbidities (e.g., hypertension and diabetes), and current medications. Adjusted HRs are similar to ORs and are commonly found in cohort studies. HRs compare different cohorts relative to the timing of the outcome – e.g., if subjects survived or when subjects died.

Reading the results

Q6 *How was the sample characterized?*

The study population consisted of 122,007 patients. Table 7.1 in the article divided the population across demographic and health variables (e.g., comorbidities and smoking status), and along the five CRF performance groups. The study reported an increase in comorbidities from low to high CRF performance groups. These comorbidities were later adjusted to refine the association between CRF and mortality more clearly.

Q7 *Which relationships were reported to be statistically significant (or not)? and*

Q8 *How strong were the relationships?*

The study tracked five cohorts to explore differences in all-cause mortality over a 24-year period. Comparisons were made between pairs of cohorts, using HRs to estimate the strength of the relations. The leftmost column in Table 7.3 shows which CRF cohorts are being compared. The lowest CRF cohort served as the reference cohort against which others were compared. The middle column presents adjusted HRs along with the 95% CIs associated with each estimate. The rightmost column indicates whether the groups being compared are significantly different with respect to mortality.

Differences between cohorts were all statistically significant $p < 0.001$. Point estimates shown in the middle column suggest a progressive increase in the aHR at higher and higher levels of CRF. Comparing the low to below-average CRF group shows an aHR of

TABLE 7.3 Risk-adjusted all-Cause mortality across 5 cohorts stratified by cardiorespiratory fitness

CRF group comparison	aHR (95% CI)*	p-value
Low CRF	1.00 (referent)	
Below average	1.95 (1.86–2.14)	<0.001
Above average	2.75 (2.61–2.89)	<0.001
High	3.90 (3.67–4.14)	<0.001
Elite	5.04 (4.10–6.20)	<0.001

Adapted from "Risk-adjusted All-Cause Mortality, Comorbidities and Performance Groups". Data from [3].

* HRs are adjusted for age, gender, smoking, and various comorbidities.

1.95 – 95% higher for the low compared to the below-average CRF group. For the elite CRF group, the adjusted HR was 5.04. The average risk of mortality for the low CRF group is 5.04 times higher compared to the elite CRF group.

Though not definitive, this evidence suggests a dose-response between cardiorespiratory fitness and all-cause mortality. Further, the article identified a significant reduction in all-cause mortality was found among elite, compared to high CRF cohorts (aHR = 1.29, p = 0.02). This also offers evidence that there is no upper limit on the beneficial effects of aerobic fitness.

Reading the discussion

Q9 *What were the strengths and limitations of the study?*

The study provided strong evidence of a dose-response relationship between CRF and mortality – higher CRF is associated with lower all-cause mortality – and reinforced evidence provided in other studies. Moreover, this reduction in all-cause mortality was shown in the elite cohort, suggesting that health benefits continue at higher and higher levels of CRF. The study fulfilled a major aim in showing that the effects of CRF did not plateau at high and elite levels of CRF levels.

The article identifies limitations associated with the classification of CRF into five levels, since no clear consensus has been reached regarding CRF measurement. This poses a challenge, particularly in comparing the results of this study to those of others that gauge CRF in a different way.

Importantly, not all potential confounding variables that might affect the relationship between CRF and all-cause mortality were controlled. The study was able to adjust for several comorbidities and some other variables, but other unmeasured variables – e.g., socioeconomic status (SES) and race/ethnicity – were not included in the analysis. For instance, SES was not included in health records so could not be extracted and adjusted for. It is entirely plausible or even likely that SES affects both CRF and mortality, thereby confounding the results.

Finally, of the observational study designs, cohort studies are most effective in supporting a causal linkage between exposure and outcome (see Box 7.3). The dose-response relationship reported in this study, along with other studies that identify biological mechanisms that connect CRF to overall fitness and longevity, suggest a broader causal relationship.

BOX 7.3   COHORT STUDIES AND CAUSALITY

We suggest that the term "association" be used to characterize a relationship between outcome and exposure reported in observational studies. Reference to "causal" associations may be used for relationships found in an experiment. Control over study variables is much greater in experiments, which increases the ability to rule out alternative explanations for the association. Yet, consistently strong "dose-response" relationships from several cohort designs, especially those with a sound explanation of the link between exposure and outcome, surely are suggestive of a causal association.

Q10 What were the implications of the study for research and practice?

The article provides strong evidence supporting the effects of CRF on all-cause mortality. Cardiorespiratory fitness is considered as a modifiable risk factor that can affect how long we live. How modifiable CRF is will likely vary, depending on the everyday circumstances in which people live – some circumstances are more conducive to behavior change than others. Health professionals would do well to take these variable circumstances into account to recommend realistic ways to improve CRF.

Example 7.4 Analytically reading a hybrid study

Hybrid designs employ two research designs in a single primary study. For instance, qualitative and quantitative designs might complement each other in single "mixed-methods" study (see Example 9.2). Researchers also combine advantages of case-control and cohort designs in a single study. For instance, researchers select a subset of cases from a larger cohort, match them with controls, and compare the two in terms of exposures – the case-control design is nested within a larger cohort study.

In the example below, researchers combine a case-control and cohort designs to study (a) differences between matched ACL-injured cases and uninjured controls in terms of prior "playing style" and (b) differences between cases and controls post-ACL reconstruction in terms of player performance.

Title. "Tendency of Driving to the Basket Is Associated with Increased Risk of Anterior Cruciate Ligament Tears in National Basketball Association Players: A Cohort Study" [4].

Inspectional reading

Readers will have answered the first two analytical questions based on the title, abstract, and introduction. The study explores the association between style of play and anterior cruciate ligament (ACL) injury among NBA players (a case-control design), and between ACL reconstruction (ACLR) and subsequent performance (a cohort design). The twofold hypothesis suggests that both designs will be used, expecting that

1 players' tendency to drive to the basket will be associated with ACL tears, and
2 players' performance will decline after ACL reconstruction.

Testing these hypotheses requires a two-part, hybrid research design (see Figure 7.1). The first hypothesis would be tested by comparing ACL-injured NBA players (cases) to matched, uninjured controls in terms of previous exposure – i.e., driving tendency. The second hypothesis would be tested by comparing performance statistics among cases after ACLR to their matched controls.

Reading the methods

Q3 What inclusion/exclusion criteria did the study use to select the sample?

For this study, secondary, publicly available data on NBA player statistics from 1980 to 2017 were aggregated and analyzed. Forty-nine (49) demographics (e.g., year and age), anthropometric (e.g., height and BMI), and performance statistics (e.g., points, rebounds,

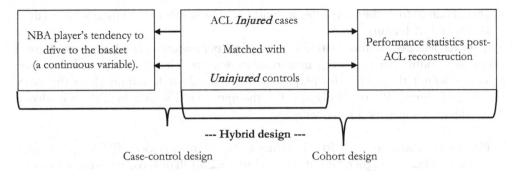

FIGURE 7.1   Hybrid case-control – cohort design.

assists) were collected. Using these metrics, fifty (50) ACL-injured players (cases) were each matched (based on metrics, age, and year of play) with 100 non-injured players (controls) in terms of the playing style (e.g., driving tendency).

Q4 How valid and reliable were the variable measures?

The hypothesis suggests that the tendency to drive would be associated with ACL injury. Driving tendency was measured as drives per minute while controlling for minutes played and utilization. Another hypothesis suggests that performance would decline after ACL injury. Besides assessing how driving tendency was altered post-injury, performance was measured in terms of the rate of 3-point attempts.

Q5 How were the data analyzed?

The study expected that exposure to driving tendency (i.e., players who tended to drive more) would be for cases than controls. It is further expected that performance would decline more for cases post-ACL reconstruction (ACLR) and for controls. Comparisons between cases and controls in terms of driving tendency were made using paired t tests. Comparisons between cases and controls in terms of performance after ACLR also used paired z tests. The alpha level for statistical significance was set to $p < 0.05$.

Reading the results

Q6 How was the sample characterized?

The first table in the article presented comparisons between 50 injured cases and 100 matched, uninjured controls. Across all metrics (age, year, performance metrics), no significant differences were found – all p-values reported as ≥ 0.05. This suggests a confidence that cases and matched controls were comparable across numerous performance dimensions, including driving tendency.

Q7 Which relationships were reported to be statistically significant (or not)?

In describing the relationship between drive tendency and ACL injury, the article reports

> Players who had an ACL injury in the NBA were observed to have a significantly greater career-average drive tendency compared with controls ($p =.047$) [4].

Thus, findings from the study offer support to the view of an association between drive tendency and ACL injury.

Drive tendency is a numeric variable (i.e., drives per minute) – i.e., frequency of drives exists on a continuous scale with numerous increments. The study reported that drive tendency did not affect injury for players up to 1.0 standard deviations above the mean, inclusive of about 84% of all players. For the upper 16% with a high-drive tendency, ACL injury rates increased incrementally.

> Players with career-average drive tendency ≥ 1 standard deviation (SD) above the mean had a significantly higher rate of ACL injury (5.2%) than those with career-average drive tendency < 1 SD (2.7%) (p = .026; relative risk, 1.9) [4].

In short, a statistically significant difference in ACL injury was observed for players assessed at 1.0 SD or more above the mean compared to those below that threshold (p = 0.026).

The cohort design portion of this hybrid study compared performance outcomes for players injured cases after ACL reconstruction (ACLR) to the uninjured controls. The study reported no significant differences in several performance indicators between cases and controls – total points (p = 0.164), minutes (p = 0.237), drive tendency (p = 0.152) and 3-point attempts (p = 0.508). Thus, the evidence did not support the second hypothesis that the performance would decline after ACLR.

Q8 How strong were the relationships?

The study identified an increase in the relative risk (RR) of ACL injury between players above or below the 1 SD threshold (RR = 1.9, p = 0.026). Otherwise, the study did not report statistics on the strength of the effect of driving tendency on ACL injury.

Reading the discussion

Q9 What were the strengths and limitations of the study?

This article identified an association between driving tendency and ACL injury (among NBA players). It makes sense intuitively that the tendency to slash and cut on a basketball court would put more force on knees, subjecting them to higher risk of injury compared to players whose role principally favors shooting.

The study also compared performance of injured cases and uninjured controls in the years after ACLR, expecting that the injury would degrade performance. Although changes in performance were observed during the years after injury, the changes might be due to normal aging or other unrelated factors. No significant differences in performance were found between cases and controls.

Findings from this observational study showed associations between driving tendency and ACL injury. Yet this does not mean that driving tendency *causes* ACL injury, at least not directly. While several variables were controlled for assessing the association between drive tendency and injury, the case control design cannot control all possible variables that might contribute to injury risk. Hence, the article cautions against making a causal claim about the association between drive tendency and ACL injury.

The study population was of elite athletes. These athletes are much more physically equipped to compete at the highest level, and train regularly to maintain or increase fitness levels. The results from this unique population might not apply to basketball players, at lower levels, to younger, developing players, or to female basketball players.

Q10 *What were the implications of the study for research and practice?*

Drive tendency serves as an imperfect proxy for the biomechanical variables that underlie ACL strain and injury. The article recommends further research to more clearly characterize the biomechanical actions involved with driving and shooting that contribute to ACL strain and injury. Meanwhile, the study recommends using ACL tear prevention programs for high-drive tendency players.

Recap

This Chapter provides an overview of how to critically engage with peer-reviewed observational studies, incorporating examples across different study designs—cross-sectional, case-control, and cohort studies, as well as a hybrid design that combined case-control and cohort elements. It uses the ten analytical questions identified in Chapter 5 to activate the reading process and to guide readers in the critical assessment of observational studies.

Example 7.1 discussed is a cross-sectional study utilizing NHANES data to analyze health behaviors of American pregnant women, emphasizing the importance of understanding data collection methods, relevance to the population of interest, and the reliability of self-reported measures.

Example 7.2 explores a case-control study by the CDC on COVID-19, highlighting the utility of this design for rapidly gathering data during the pandemic and the limitations of self-reported exposure information.

Example 7.3 delves into a cohort study assessing the long-term mortality impact of cardiorespiratory fitness, demonstrating the strength of cohort studies in observing outcomes over time while also noting the potential confounders not controlled for in the study.

Example 7.4 presents a hybrid design, integrating aspects of case-control and cohort studies to examine the risk of ACL injuries among NBA players in relation to their playing style and performance post-injury. This section underscores the complexity of linking specific behaviors to injury risks and the need for targeted prevention strategies.

Each example showed the application of analytical questions to assess a study's relevance, design, data collection and analysis methods, findings, and implications. The examples help to enhance the reader's ability to identify and critically assess the strengths and limitations of observational studies to facilitate a deeper understanding of the implications of observational research for evidence-based practice.

References

1. Francis EC, Zhang L, Witrick B, Chen L. Health behaviors of American pregnant women: A cross-sectional analysis of NHANES 2007–2014. *J Public Health (Oxf)*. 2021;43(1):131–138. doi:10.1093/pubmed/fdz117.
2. Fisher KA, Tenforde MW, Feldstein LR, Lindsell CJ, Shapiro NI, Files DC. Community and close contact exposures associated with COVID-19 among symptomatic adults ≥18 years in 11 outpatient health care facilities—United States, July 2020. *MMWR Morb Mortal Wkly Rep*. 2020;69(36):1258–1264. doi:10.15585/mmwr.mm6936a5.
3. Mandsager K, Harb S, Cremer P, Phelan D, Nissen SE, Jaber W. Association of cardiorespiratory fitness with long-term mortality among adults undergoing exercise treadmill testing. *JAMA Netw Open*. 2018;1(6):e183605. doi:10.1001/jamanetworkopen.2018.3605.
4. Schultz BJ, Thomas KA, Cinque M, Harris JD, Maloney WJ, Abrams GD. Tendency of driving to the basket is associated with increased risk of anterior cruciate ligament tears in National Basketball Association players: A cohort study. *Orthop J Sports Med*. 2021;9(11):2325967121 1052953. doi:10.1177/23259671211052953.

8

UNDERSTANDING EXPERIMENTAL DESIGNS

Overview of experimental designs

Readers have seen that observational studies identify associations between exposures and health outcomes, as they are observed in their natural settings. With varying degrees of precision and confidence, observational studies help us predict the likelihood of a health outcome occurring. This can inform steps to be taken to encourage positive outcomes and discourage negative ones.

In contrast, experimental studies seek to determine the causes of health outcomes through the applications of controlled interventions – manipulating variables and observing their effects. Thus, the hallmark of an experiment is its attempt to control variables to isolate causes and effects.

Experiments that occur in a basic science microbiology lab have virtually complete control over experimental conditions and are well suited to isolating and assessing causal mechanisms. Experimental control in animal research can be substantial as well, but there are ethical limits to the conditions researchers will expose animals to (especially mammals) for the sake of science. Experimental control over what researchers may expose human subjects to is even more limited, both practically and ethically.

Here we describe three general types of experimental designs described here – natural experiments, quasi-experiments, and true experiments. We introduce the discussion, however, by describing a pre-experimental design – the single-group pretest-posttest design. These designs differ in the extent of control experimental studies have over variables and the ability to establish causal relationships.

Experimental control

Experimental designs differ in terms of control over the research process. As shown in Table 8.1, the researcher's control over (1) the administration of the intervention (2) the groups being compared, and (3) the assignment of subjects to groups (random or not random) serves to differentiate types of experimental designs.

DOI: 10.4324/9781003595663-10

TABLE 8.1 Experimental control and research designs: single-group pretest-posttest, natural, quasi-, and true experiments

Design/ feature	Cohort designs	Experimental designs*			
		Single-group pretest-posttest	Natural Exp.	Quasi-Exp.	True Exp.
Administer intervention	No	Yes	No, natural occurrence	Yes	Yes
Random assignment	No	Not applicable	"As if" random	No	Yes
Major comparison	Between exposure groups	Change in outcome pre- and post-intervention	Between experimental groups	Between experimental groups	Between experimental groups
Examples	Associations between diet and longevity	Effect of new T2D therapy	Effects of minimum wage on well-being	Effects of signage on food choices	Effects of mindfulness on anxiety

* Pretest-Posttest designs are a common subtype of "pre-experimental" designs. In natural experiments, the assumption "as if random" refers to the role chance is said to play with respect to being affected by a natural event or policy. The validity of this assumption is tested by comparing groups across key variables.

Control over the intervention

Observational studies do not introduce intervention and, therefore, do not control which groups are exposed. This is also the case for natural experiments, which assess the widespread impact of natural events such as fires, floods, or pandemics. A new law or policy is similar to "natural" events in that their introduction has widespread effects (see Example 9.1).

Because of the sudden, widespread effects the exposure is considered the "intervention" in a natural experiment, even though the researchers do not control or manipulate it. This distinguishes natural experiments from the other, more common experimental designs where the researcher controls the administration of the intervention. This experimental control enables the intervention to be replicated, refined, and tested to characterize a causal link more precisely to the health outcome.

Comparisons

Quantitative studies vary regarding the comparisons they make. In the case of single-group pretest-posttest designs, researchers administer the intervention to all participants and examine outcomes before and after (changes). In this case, as a single-group design, there are no group comparisons – outcomes are measured before and after the intervention is administered and any changes are identified.

Without a comparison group, however, the single-group design cannot rule out other possible explanations of any changes that are observed. For instance, observed changes in outcomes might be attributed to natural changes that occur over time due to maturation or as side-effects of external events (e.g., pandemics). Observed change might also be explained by the statistical tendency for unusually high or low values to migrate toward the mean in subsequent measurements. Observed change might be due to change in performance that can occur with repeated testing (see Appendix B on maturation, regression to the mean, and test-retest bias).

These biases confound the interpretation of the effects of the intervention on the outcome. This limitation is remedied in natural, quasi-, and true experiments where two or more experimental groups are exposed to the intervention and their effects are compared (see Box 8.1).

BOX 8.1 EXPERIMENTAL GROUPS

The term 'experimental groups' generally refers to all groups in an experiment. This may include just two groups – an experimental group that receives the intervention and a control group that does not. However, experimental groups may vary in terms of the types or levels of the intervention each one receives. For instance, a study might compare the effects of different doses of a dietary supplement, different diets, or different workout programs. Typically, the main control group might receive the "usual and customary" treatment intervention that serves as a baseline for comparison. In randomized controlled trials, an experimental group might receive a placebo – a sham treatment that contains no therapeutic agent and is used to assess the psychological effects of receiving the intervention.

Random assignment

Random assignment refers to the process of allocating research subjects to different experimental groups based purely on chance. The ability to randomly assign subjects to experimental groups implies a level of experimental control that characterizes a "true" experiment.

In contrast, some natural experiments assume that exposure to an external event mimics random assignment. For instance, residents to adjacent streets are, on average, similar. A tornado devastates homes on First Street but misses homes on Second Street. Exposure to the intervention could be said to have occurred "as if" at random. The validity of this assumption is to be assessed.

Quasi-experimental designs resemble "true" experiments in terms of controlling the administration of the intervention. With quasi-experiments, however, participants who volunteer will receive the intervention, while comparison group of non-volunteers do not. Pre-existing differences between the groups are uncontrolled and confound the results.

Random assignment serves to balance the distribution of confounder variables evenly across groups, so their effects on the outcome cancel each other out. Thus, experimental control limits the risk of biases and helps isolate the effects of the intervention on health outcomes.

Single-group, pretest-posttest designs

Single-group, pretest-posttest designs (aka, the "one-shot" pre-experimental design) assess changes in the outcome before and after the intervention is administered (see Box 8.2). Pretest-posttest designs are often used to initially test an intervention to determine

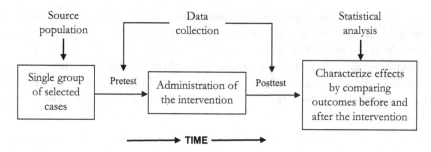

FIGURE 8.1   Single-group pretest-posttest design.

whether it is safe and feasible to administer and whether it produces positive health effects. As shown in Figure 8.1, observations are recorded for a single group before and after exposure to the intervention. This before-after comparison describes the change that results from exposure to the intervention.

BOX 8.2   PRE-EXPERIMENTAL DESIGNS

The single-group pre-experimental design compares the same group before and after the intervention is administered. A "static-group" pre-experimental design compares the outcome of two groups – one that received an intervention and another that did not. Outcome differences are assumed to have resulted from the intervention.

For instance, a 2-week, curriculum-based mindfulness intervention was introduced to first-year college students to test the effects on psychological distress, using measures of depression, anxiety, and stress. Researchers observed a significant change in distress pre- and post-intervention ($p = 0.01$). The intervention showed promise, but without a comparison group, the study could not rule out plausible alternative explanations – e.g., natural growth and maturation of college students, adjustment to college life, unusually high scores on distress naturally regressed toward a mean score [1].

Another study showed similar promise for improving motor function among people with Parkinson's disease. Sampled patients were exposed to a low-resistance, interval bicycling intervention and, over several weeks, showed significant improvement in function. Nonetheless, without a comparison group researchers could not rule out plausible alternative explanations for improvement – e.g., placebo effects, test-retest bias, mitigation of the ailment due to other factors [2].

Strengths and limitations of single-group pretest-posttest studies

Single-group pretest-posttest designs are useful for initially testing an intervention to determine its feasibility and effectiveness. The design enables researchers to measure changes in the outcome before and after the intervention was administered. The design costs less to implement and promising interventions can then be refined and retested and perhaps tested with a comparison group in a "true" experiment.

A major limitation of pretest-posttest designs is the lack of a comparison group. This omission means several extraneous factors might have affected the result – e.g., cases naturally change over time (maturation), test results may improve through repetition, and, over time, results regress toward the mean (Appendix B). Subjects dropping out due to issues related to the intervention will also skew results and limit the generalizability of the findings.

Natural experiments

Natural experiments are like cohort studies in that researchers do not control exposure to an intervention but instead observe the effects of the exposures over time. However, natural experiments differ from cohort studies in that the exposure is often sudden and produces system-wide effects. These are "natural" events such as famine, hurricanes, or pandemics. They also include large-scale human-created events like a new law expanding Medicaid benefits or a mandate requiring facemasks to be worn in public schools. Though researchers do not administer the intervention, they can observe changes in outcomes before and after the event occurred to assess its effects (see Figure 8.2).

Strictly speaking, researchers do not control who is or is not exposed to the intervention. For instance, a tornado might strike one row of houses but miss a second row, seemingly at random. By assuming that there are no pre-existing differences between the two rows, assignment of subjects can be said to have occurred "as if" at random. The assumption of "as if" or "quasi" randomization can be tested by comparing the two groups to evaluate their equivalence before the event occurred.

For instance, to investigate the effects of a minimum wage law on mental health, researchers compared depressive symptoms among low-wage workers before and after the introduction of a national minimum wage [3]. All low-wage workers in the UK were eligible for an increase, but some firms did not comply. "As-if" randomization would assume that there are no pre-existing differences between low-wage workers of compliant and

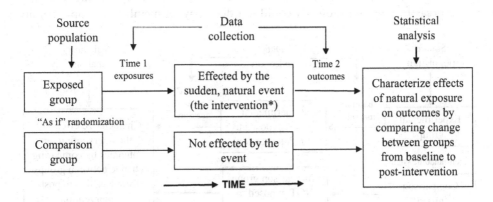

*NOTE: The intervention is an event or process that has widespread effects but is not administered by the research team.

FIGURE 8.2   The structure of the natural experiment.

non-complaint firms. The plausibility of the assumption can be assessed on its surface, but also by comparing group differences across covariates (see Example 9.1).

Strengths and limitations of natural experiments

Natural experiments investigate the system-wide effects of an "intervention" on an outcome, offering evidence that supports causal inferences. Natural experiments take place outside the lab and in the natural world and in this way, they resemble cohort studies. Although we may not control when and where certain natural events occur, studying them helps us understand their effects and better manage our responses. Natural experiments that assess the effects of new laws or policies also advance evidence-based discussion to inform future policies and actions.

Since the intervention cannot be controlled, natural experiments are difficult to replicate. Therefore, relationships found between exposure and outcome in a natural experiment should be consistent with findings from other studies using other designs (e.g., cohort and RCTs).

Quasi-experimental designs

Quasi-experiments differ from natural experiments in that the researcher controls the administration of the intervention to compare the change in health outcomes among experimental groups. Unlike natural experiments, quasi-experiments can be replicated and refined and tested in different populations.

The structure of quasi-experiments is shown in Figure 8.3.

In quasi-experiments researchers do not control who is and is not exposed to the intervention, and research subjects are not randomly assigned to one or another experimental group. Quasi-experiments test the intervention with volunteer participants, often relying on non-volunteers, sometimes from different source populations, to use for comparison. Thus, pre-existing differences between the groups may confound the results.

For instance, an insurance company aimed to test the effects of a breastfeeding program on breastfeeding duration but could not deny paying members the opportunity to

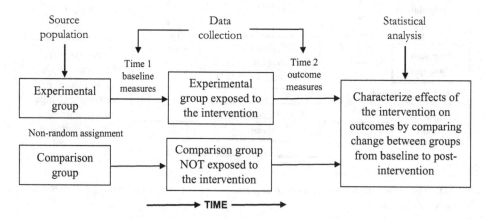

FIGURE 8.3 The structure of the quasi-experiment.

participate (it was available to everyone), nor could they compel members to participate in the program (participation was not required). The study tested the effects on volunteers who might differ in important ways from non-volunteers, and these pre-existing differences may confound the results (see Example 9.2). Quasi-experiments will assess covariates to statistically adjust for pre-existing differences, but this cannot account for numerous other unmeasured group differences that might affect the results.

Strengths and limitations of quasi-experiments

As an intervention study, the quasi-experiment may suggest a causal interpretation of the relationship between the intervention and the outcome, especially when the results point in a direction that is theoretically plausible and consistent with other studies. Moreover, unlike natural experiments, in quasi-experiments, the researcher controls the administration of the intervention, enabling the study to be replicated and the intervention refined, adapted, and tested with different populations.

Where random assignment is not practical or ethical, quasi-experiments offer an alternative way to assess the effects of an intervention on health outcomes. Further, results may reflect how an intervention works and its effects in the "real world" rather than in a more controlled setting. In this regard, results of quasi-experiments are more applicable to practice settings (see Box 8.3).

This strength is also a weakness. The lack of randomization contributes to selection bias, where pre-existing group differences confound the results. The vulnerability to confounding variables threatens the study's "internal validity" and limits the ability to make causal inferences.

BOX 8.3   ECOLOGICAL VALIDITY

Ecological validity pertains to the validity of generalizing results from the study setting to other settings. The breastfeeding program's reliance on eager volunteers may better reflect how the program might work if rolled out more widely. In contrast, results from "true" experiments conducted in artificial settings may not reflect how interventions actually operate and impact results under real-world conditions. Not all true experiments face this limitation, however. For instance, clinical trials of the COVID-19 vaccines enable subjects, once given the vaccine or a placebo, to return to their daily lives to test the vaccine's effectiveness against natural exposure to the virus.

"True" experiments

True experiments are like quasi-experiments in terms of control over the administration of the intervention. This enables interventions to be refined and retested. True experiments differ from quasi-experiments, however, in the random assignment of subjects to either an experimental or control group. The logic of the design is shown in Figure 8.4.

Random assignment involves allocating each subject to an experimental group based on chance – in effect, by flipping a coin. The larger the sample, the more confident we are

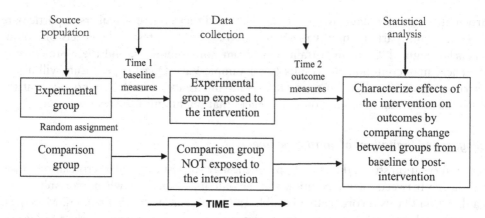

FIGURE 8.4 The structure of the true experiment.

that the process of randomization will distribute attributes evenly across all groups. This even distribution helps ensure that the groups are comparable at baseline, as potential confounding variables cancel out. If groups are equivalent at baseline, we become more confident in attributing changes in outcomes to the intervention.

For instance, to compare the effects of dietary interventions on obesity and adiposity, researchers randomly assigned 294 patients to one of three intervention groups – healthy diet guidance, Mediterranean, and green Mediterranean dietary interventions (see Example 9.3) [4]. Although all patients chose to participate in the study, they did not choose which intervention they would receive. Across twenty-plus characteristics, no significant differences were found between the groups at baseline – e.g., mean age was 51.1, 51.7, and 50.5 years ($p = 0.76$). Unmeasured differences are assumed to be randomly distributed across the groups as well. Thus, differences found after 6 months (i.e., post-intervention) could plausibly be attributed to the effects of the intervention (see Example 9.3).

Randomized controlled trials (RCTs)

Randomized controlled trials (RCTs) are considered the "gold standard" for health science research designs (see Box 8.4). Besides randomizing subjects to either an experimental or control group, RCTs may add other controls to limit the effects of potential confounders.

For instance, we know that subjects' expectations regarding the effectiveness of an intervention can have a real impact on the results – aka, the "placebo" effect. Likewise, the expectations of researchers may also influence participants' behaviors and can bias the results – e.g., the "Pygmalion" or "Rosenthal" effect (see Appendix B). To limit these effects, RCTs will conceal the allocation of the intervention from research participants or from observers or from both – a process referred to as "blinding". For instance, in a double-blind RCT designed to test a new drug, neither participant nor the researcher will know if the treatment intervention contains the active ingredient. Thus, placebo and Pygmalion effects are neutralized. For many tests of interventions, however, blinding is not possible.

BOX 8.4 PHASES OF RCTS

Pre-clinical experiments are often undertaken before a fully-fledged RCT is initiated. Testing may begin in a microbiology lab (*in vitro*) to determine antigens which might prevent or block disease from developing. Preclinical phases also include testing on animals, and then on a small number of *healthy* humans to first assess its safety, and then its efficacy. Assuming positive results, more human volunteers can be added, and the intervention can be refined to improve its efficacy and test its effects in different populations. If successful, the intervention may reach a full clinical trial phase, where larger numbers are tested for safety and effectiveness in different populations.

Crossover experimental designs

Many experimental studies use a parallel-group design where the experimental and control groups are studied in parallel, with one group exposed to the intervention while the other is not. In contrast, in crossover designs all subjects are exposed to the intervention, however, in a certain sequence.

For instance, the effects of an intervention would be tested on one group while a second group rested (e.g., as a control). After a suitable "washout" period where the effects of the intervention return to baseline levels, the groups would switch roles – group 1 would rest, and group 2 would receive the intervention. Thus, the effects of the intervention would be compared to the effects of rest for each subject.

An important advantage of crossover designs is the ability to make within-subject comparison of the effects of the interventions since each subject responds to both treatment conditions (the intervention and control). This contrasts with parallel group designs, where subjects in the intervention group are compared to and different from subjects in the control group. Since intra-subject variation is lower than between-subject variation, crossover designs benefit from more reliable measures of change. In addition, crossover designs require fewer subjects to detect statistically significant effects, reducing total costs, in terms of time, energy, and money.

One disadvantage of crossover designs is that they are not suitable for interventions that have lasting or irreversible effects. For instance, the effects of educational programs, lifestyle interventions, or vaccinations endure, making it impossible to identify a definite washout period for a crossover to occur. Thus, crossover designs are mainly used to test interventions that do not produce long-lasting or permanent effects – e.g., short-term dietary interventions, pain management programs, exercise interventions.

Strengths and limitations of true experiments

Random assignment limits the impact of confounding variables on outcomes. This reduces the risk of bias as it limits the range of plausible alternative explanations for change in the outcome. This enhances our confidence that the observed changes in the outcome were caused by the intervention.

A chief strength of the experiment is its control over the intervention and assignment of subjects to experimental groups. This strength, however, can come at a cost – results that appear under controlled conditions may not play out in the same way under real-world conditions where numerous variables interact. Experimental control sometimes reduces the applicability of the evidence in real-world settings (Box 8.3, on ecological validity).

Experiments often employ strict inclusion and exclusion criteria in the selection of participants for a study. As always, therefore, readers should carefully consider the characteristics of the sample population when contemplating how and where the results might apply. Results that apply to adolescents may not apply to elders; they may apply for men but not for women; for middle-class families but not impoverished ones. Inclusion and exclusion criteria help define for us where and to whom results may apply. It also reminds us of the importance of examining results from multiple studies on the topic to gauge its applicability to different contexts and people.

Recap

This chapter discussed the fundamental concepts and methodologies associated with experimental research designs. It suggested that experimental designs are especially useful for testing the effects of a specific intervention or manipulation on health outcomes. While observational studies improve the ability to *predict* health outcomes, testing and refining experimental interventions to improve our *control* over these outcomes.

The chapter describes three major types of experimental designs – natural experiments, quasi-experiments, and true experiments. It also briefly outlines two variants of true experiments – the randomized controlled trial (RCT) and the crossover experimental design. Experiments vary with respect to the ability to control the intervention and randomly assign research participants to experimental groups. Greater control serves to reduce research biases and to isolate the effects of the intervention on health outcomes. This control strengthens claims that observed changes in outcomes were *caused* by the intervention. Understanding how these designs differ regarding experimental control enhances our grasp of the strengths and limits of research findings, along with their implications for evidence-based practice.

References

1. Glena VS, Mushquash AR, Gotwals JK, Sinden KE, Pearson ES. "Staying in the present moment is important": Examining the impact of a short-term classroom-based mindfulness intervention among first-year students. *J Am Coll Health*. 2022:1–10. doi:10.1080/07448481.2022.2155057.
2. Uygur M, Bellumori M, Knight CA. Effects of a low-resistance, interval bicycling intervention in Parkinson's disease. *Physiother Theory Pract*. 2017;33(12):897–904. doi:10.1080/09593985.2017.1359868.
3. Reeves A, McKee M, Mackenbach J, Whitehead M, Stuckler D. Introduction of a national minimum wage reduced depressive symptoms in low-wage workers: A quasi-natural experiment in the UK. *Health Econ*. 2017;26(5):639–655. doi:10.1002/hec.3336.
4. Tsaban G, Meir AY, Rinott E, Zelicha H, Kaplan A, Shalev A, et al. The effect of green Mediterranean diet on cardiometabolic risk: A randomised controlled trial. *Heart*. 2021;107(13):1054–1061. doi:10.1136/heartjnl-2020-317802.

9
ANALYTICALLY READING EXPERIMENTAL

This chapter provides three examples to illustrate the process of analytically reading peer-reviewed studies that use natural, quasi, and true experimental designs. The quasi-experimental study examines the effects of an educational intervention designed to promote breastfeeding. The true experiment tests the effects of a dietary intervention designed to reduce metabolic risk.

We start with a natural experiment that assesses the effects of national minimum wage legislation on depressive symptoms among low-wage workers. The intervention is system-wide, but some low-wage workers received the wage increase while others did not. This study tests the as-if randomization assumption in addition to the change in depression scores before and after the introduction of a new minimum wage.

Example 9.1   A natural experiment

Title: "Introduction of a national minimum wage reduced depressive symptoms in low-wage workers: a quasi-natural experiment in the UK" [1].

Inspectional reading

Readers will already have answered the first two analytical questions based on the title, abstract, and introduction.

Q1 Is the study relevant?

Q2 What study design was used?

By inspecting the title, you will see what the study is about – i.e., the effects of the introduction of a national minimum wage on depressive symptoms of low-wage workers in the UK. The "intervention" in this natural experiment was the introduction of legislation that raised the minimum wage.

DOI: 10.4324/9781003595663-11

The abstract provides the study's storyline. The study used longitudinal data from the British Household Panel Survey (BHPS) and a 12-item General Health Questionnaire to assess mental health of low-wage workers before and after the legislation was introduced. The study analyzed depressive symptoms of low-wage workers before and after the legislation was introduced. While other studies examined the various effects of the minimum wage legislation, none had explored the effects of such legislation on health. The aim of the study was to test the effects of increasing wages and mental health.

Reading the methods

Q3 *What inclusion/exclusion criteria did the study use to select the sample?*

Readers will examine how subjects were selected – the inclusion and exclusion criteria. The study used secondary data, drawing from 5,500 households (circa 10,000 individuals) responding to the ongoing panel study – the British Household Panel Survey (BHPS). Households were stratified and randomly selected; details of the sampling process were described elsewhere. Noteworthy is that the same individuals were interviewed in successive waves, which is essential for any study that examines change over time.

The study excluded men and women under 22 years to whom the law would not fully apply and persons over 59 who were eligible for pensions. It divided the sample into those who received a wage increase and those who did not, either because some earned slightly more than minimum wage (control group 1) or because their firm did not comply with the legislation (control group 2). Readers will consider how pre-existing group differences that affect health might challenge the assumption of as-if randomization and confound the interpretation of the effects of the legislation. Table 1 of the Results section will supply this information.

Q4 *How valid and reliable were the variable measures?*

This study used the UK's General Health Questionnaire (GHQ) as the principal source of outcome variables in the study. The study sourced other studies to attest to the reliability of the GHQ mental health scale.

The study also used the BHPS to assess aspects of physical health – e.g., blood pressure, smoking, and hearing loss. Hearing loss is used as a red flag "falsification test" – an irrelevant, "placebo" variable used to assess the validity of the method. Since hearing loss usually occurs gradually and is unlikely to be influenced by the legislation, detecting substantial hearing loss would signal a problem with the validity of the methods. Detecting no hearing change would enhance our confidence in them.

Wages were self-reported as gross monthly income divided by the number of hours worked. Aware of possible biases in self-reported measures, the study checked their validity by selecting a subset of the self-reports and verifying them against actual pay slips. Covariates were assessed to adjust for key characteristics of the study populations – e.g., age, sex, social class, education.

Q5 *How were the data analyzed?*

To estimate the effect of the wage legislation, the study estimated the change in general health and depression scores before and after its enactment, adjusting for covariates.

Change scores for the intervention group were compared to each of the control groups. Group change scores would then be compared to determine if differences were significant and to measure the strength of the effects.

Reading the results

Q6 How was the sample characterized?

Readers will locate Table 1 in the article, which describes attributes of the selected population – sociodemographic, health, housing, and employment ($n = 279$). The table also identified the p-value to assess pre-existing differences between experimental groups. This serves to identify possible confounding variables and how well the as-if randomization assumption is supported.

 The table showed no significant differences between the intervention and the control groups across a range of covariates. Since no significant between-group differences were found across these variables, the study's as-if random assumption is supported.

Q7 Which relationships were reported to be statistically significant (or not)?

The results reported in Table II of the article showed a statistically significant difference between the intervention and control group 1 in terms of change in GHQ scores – $p = 0.025$ – and self-reported anxiety/depression – $p = 0.016$. It is highly unlikely that the difference found resulted from chance, thereby supporting a claim that decline in GHQ scores was due to the minimum wage increase.

Q8 How strong were the relationships?

While the relationship between the intervention and GHQ scores is not likely to be due to chance, readers will also seek to know how strong the effect is. The article presents an estimate of the improvement in total GHQ scores – how much did the legislation affect change in GHQ scores? The study reports an improvement of 0.70 in GHQ scores before and after the legislation, and a 0.23 decline in scores for control group 1 – a net difference in scores of 0.93. This approximates an improvement of 0.373 of a standard deviation.

 For most readers, an improvement of 0.373 standard deviations may mean little in terms of the effect of the legislation. The article, however, translates the number in more meaningful terms. The improvement would be "comparable in magnitude to the effect size estimated for antidepressants ... on depressive symptoms" [1, p. 644].

Reading the discussion

Q9 What were the strengths and limitations of the study?

The article suggests several characteristics of the study that support a causal interpretation of the association between the enactment of minimum wage legislation and improved mental health. Although random assignment of subjects to experimental groups was not possible, the assumption of as-if randomization remains largely supported by the data – intervention and control groups show no significant difference across a range of variables. Results also show a clinically significant effect size of minimum wage increases on GHQ scores to be equivalent to antidepressants. These results also align with findings from other studies that show a negative association between wage increases and financial strain and depression, offering an important contribution to our understanding of the effects of wages, financial strain, and the health of low-wage workers.

Although the experimental and control groups did not differ significantly, some selection bias may remain. For instance, the effects of working conditions for non-compliant firms are not entirely eliminated (control group 2). Although the two groups did not differ significantly in terms of job satisfaction, other characteristics of working conditions were not captured by satisfaction measures that may affect health. For instance, those working for non-compliant firms may be less well organized, and certain characteristics of their employers may be detrimental to mental health (although pre-intervention job satisfaction scores were comparable to other groups).

Study data are from surveys from 1998 to 1999 and it seems reasonable to question the relevance of these findings for today. What historical events or developments might have intervened since that time to diminish or increase the effects of financial strain on mental health? While this remains an open question, the article discussed the consistency of their findings with findings from others, suggesting minimum wage legislation would reduce distress or elevate mental health.

Q10 *What were the implications of the study for research and practice?*

Readers will consider the larger implications of the study for research, policy, and practice. The substantial impact of wage increases on employee mental health, especially for lower paid workers, might be taken seriously by employers and policy makers. In the US where health insurance is often tied to employment, wage increases might lower the overall costs of health care by decreasing the need for various physical and mental health services. Improved morale might also translate into fewer medical leave days while, potentially, advancing the productivity of workers. Public health professionals and policy advocates might also point to evidence from this and other studies to advocate for the health benefits of higher wages.

Example 9.2   A quasi-experiment

Title: "The effect of a breastfeeding support programme on breastfeeding duration and exclusivity: a quasi-experiment" [2].

Inspectional reading

Based on the title, abstract, and introduction you will already have answered the first two analytical questions. By inspecting the title, you will note that the article describes a quasi-experiment, that the main outcomes are breastfeeding duration and exclusivity, and that the intervention is a breastfeeding support program (BSP). As a quasi-experiment, participants were not randomly assigned to experimental groups. The BSP was open to volunteers, who, we later learn, differ in important ways from non-volunteers.

This selection bias confounds the interpretation of the effects of the BSP intervention. Readers will be alert to how the study analyzes and adjusts for these differences in the statistical analysis.

The Introduction describes the importance of breastfeeding for the health of infants and mothers. It also provides the theoretical approach that underlies and informs the BSP– i.e., the theory of planned behavior (TPB). It suggests that research that assesses the effectiveness of TPB-informed interventions is lacking. Thus, the study aims to examine the effects of a TPB-informed breastfeeding support program (BSP) on breastfeeding duration and exclusivity.

Reading the methods

Q3 What inclusion/exclusion criteria did the study use to select the sample?

In this study, the BSP intervention was made available by a Dutch health insurance company to anyone who wished to access it. The BSP intervention group consisted of volunteers who wished to take part in the program. The comparison group consisted of pregnant women recruited in other primary health care facilities and who expressed an intention to breastfeed and who completed an enrollment form.

The absence of random assignment alerts one to the potential for selection biases that could produce pre-existing group differences that might confound the results. Volunteers who wish to partake in the BSP intervention might be more eager, open, and able to breastfeed than are pregnant women who did not or could not volunteer. Pre-existing group differences are at risk to confound the results of the study. Several covariates may be assessed to determine this risk and to statistically adjust for group differences.

Q4 How valid and reliable were the variable measures?

The exposure – i.e., the BSP intervention – was informed by the theory of planned behavior. Based on the TPB, the BSP program attempts to influence mothers' attitudes, subject norms, and behavior. The article described the timing, delivery, and key elements of the six lactation consultations that constituted the intervention program. Periodic measures were taken for the control group, but otherwise the group received no alternative intervention.

Both experimental groups completed a pretest-posttest questionnaire used to assess the major dependent variables – breastfeeding duration and exclusivity – along with major covariates. The post-test questionnaire asked three questions designed to measure the duration and exclusivity of breastfeeding as the main outcome variables – the baby's age (in months) when breast milk ceased, when artificial feeding began, and when solid food was first received. These are critical outcome variables. The measures do not appear to have been used in prior studies or systematically tested for their validity or reliability. They also relied on self-reports, which may be subject to recall or social desirability biases (see Appendix B). Assessing the validity and reliability of how breastfeeding duration and exclusivity were measured in the study relies mainly on its apparent or "face" validity.

The questionnaires also measured 45 covariates that prior research indicated can influence breastfeeding practices. These covariates include several psychosocial variables, demographic attributes, and biomedical variables. These would be used to identify pre-existing differences between the experimental and control groups and to enable statistical adjustments to be made in the analysis.

Q5 How were the data analyzed?

The study compared experimental groups across 45 covariates to identify any significant pre-existing differences that might confound the results. Adjusting for these covariates, a hazard ratio (HR) was used to compare the experimental groups in terms of breastfeeding duration and exclusivity.

Reading the results

Q6 How was the sample characterized?

Table 1 in the article shows comparisons between the BSP and the control group across several key variables, using p-values to indicate significant pre-existing differences. For instance, compared to the control group, mothers in the BSP group saw themselves as having less control over breastfeeding ($p = 0.045$), were more likely to be first-time mothers ($p = 0.039$), and planned to work more hours ($p = 0.041$). These qualities would tend to depress breastfeeding duration and exclusivity in the BSP group compared to the control group. On the other hand, mothers in the BSP groups were, on average, more highly educated ($p = 0.002$), which might counter these effects and favor breastfeeding.

Both conflicting tendencies could skew the results in unknown ways. Although these differences are statistically adjusted for after the fact, the adjustments depend on measures that are already imperfect and cannot account for numerous unmeasured differences between groups that confound the results.

Q7 Which relationships were reported to be statistically significant (or not)?

The comparison of the intervention and control groups in terms of the duration and exclusivity of breastfeeding found significant differences between BSP and control groups.

> The effect of the BSP on survival rates for any breastfeeding was significant while controlling for differences between the two groups at baseline (HR = 0.34, $p < 0.001$ [95% CI =0.18–0.61]) [2].

A similar, statistically significant difference between the two groups in terms of breastfeeding exclusivity was also found ($p < 0.001$). The differences remained after adjusting for pre-existing differences between the groups. There is a very low probability that observed differences occurred by chance. The effects of the BSP intervention on breastfeeding were statistically significant.

Q8 *How strong were the relationships?*

The study used adjusted hazard ratios to estimate the size of the effects (Appendix F). In this example, the aHR for the intervention group relative to the non-intervention group was significantly below 1.0, both for breastfeeding duration (aHR = 0.340, CI = 0.18–0.61) and for exclusivity (aHR = 0.458, CI = 0.29–0.72).

The aHR suggests that women in the BSP intervention group were less likely to end breastfeeding or exclusive breastfeeding. In fact, an aHR estimate of 0.340 suggests that, during the time of the study, breastfeeding cessation was 66% less likely to occur in the BSP group compared to the control group. Similarly, the cessation of exclusive breast-feeding was estimated to be over half as likely (aHR=0.458) to occur in the BSP group compared to the comparison group.

Reading the discussion

Q9 *What were the strengths and limitations of the study?*

Discussion sections discuss how study results fit with results from other studies and the contribution of the results to the broader evidence on the topic. This study's find-ings "…are in line with findings from systematic reviews and meta-analyses showing the breastfeeding promotion interventions can indeed effectively increase breastfeeding rates". Moreover, the findings support the Theory of Planned Behavior (TPB) on which the intervention was based, suggesting that the BSP likely has broader application.

The study identified several pre-existing differences in the comparison groups that may confound the interpretation of the findings. The groups differed significantly across mul-tiple variables (e.g., education level, first-time mothers) that other studies have shown to produce countervailing effects on breastfeeding. Although the study statistically adjusted for several covariates, unmeasured differences could not be accounted for in the analysis. In the end, it is difficult to know how much of the variation in breastfeeding duration and exclusivity can be attributed to the BSP program as opposed to pre-existing differences between the intervention and comparison groups.

Second, analytic readers will also be cautious about generalizing from these findings to other populations. The BSP intervention group was more highly educated than the com-parison group – 92.4% compared to 68.1%. It is possible that the intervention would be less successful among populations with less education or with a low propensity for participation.

Q10 *What were the implications of the study for research and practice?*

Practitioners wanting to increase the duration and exclusivity of breastfeeding would be encouraged by the findings of the BSP. Grounded in a broader theory, it might be adapted to various other settings and populations. Such programs might be most valu-able in areas where breastfeeding rates are low. This study illustrates one of many that practitioners might examine to assess how best to increase the duration and exclusivity of breastfeeding.

Example 9.3 A true experiment

Title: "The effect of green Mediterranean diet on cardiometabolic risk; a randomised controlled trial" [3].

Inspectional reading

As the title reads, this example illustrates a true experiment, an RCT. The main intervention is a green Mediterranean diet, and the main outcome is cardiometabolic risk.

From the abstract, readers learn that three dietary groups were compared with respect to cardiometabolic risk (e.g., weight loss). The three experimental groups were: (1) the health dietary guidance (HDG) group, (2) a traditional Mediterranean (MED) diet group, and (3) the green MED diet group, which included lower intake of red meat, increased consumption of plants, polyphenols, green tea. The effects of the green MED diet on cardiometabolic risk were favorable.

Reading the methods

Q3 What inclusion/exclusion criteria did the study use to select the sample?

The study sample included employees in an "isolated workplace" – i.e., a nuclear research center in Israel. Adults over age 30 with abdominal obesity or abnormal lipid levels (dyslipidemia) were recruited for the study. In a parallel group experimental design, recruits were randomly assigned to one of three intervention groups – HDG, MED, or green MED.

Q4 How valid and reliable were the variable measures?

The three experimental groups were provided different lunches. The HDG group received health-promotion guidance for physical activity and for achieving a healthy diet. The MED group received guidance on physical activity and guidance on a low-calorie, traditional Mediterranean diet (e.g., fish, poultry, vegetables, nuts). The green MED group received similar health-promotion guidance, along with a diet richer in plants and polyphenols, green tea, and other plant-based foods.

Change pre- and post-intervention would be assessed and the groups compared with respect to various measures of cardiometabolic risk (e.g., BP, weight, waist circumference, cholesterol, fasting insulin). The study used mostly standard, clinical measures, though details surrounding their validity and reliability were not supplied.

Q5 How were the data analyzed?

Readers will identify statistics used to compare each group in terms of cardiometabolic changes. For instance, weight (in kilograms) and waist circumference (in centimeters) are continuous variables so ANOVA procedures would be used. The study used paired t-tests to evaluate how measures for individuals in each group changed before and after the intervention. It used an analysis of variance (ANOVA) to determine if differences in cardiometabolic change among groups were statistically significant. The study used chi squared tests (χ^2) to evaluate differences between categorical variables.

Reading the results

Q6 How was the sample characterized?

To understand baseline characteristics of groups and group differences, readers will, again, look to Table 1 in the Results section. Each group included 98 participants (total $n = 294$).

The Table identified baseline characteristics of each group, along with the p-values to identify significant group differences. Over 30 characteristics were assessed – e.g., age, weight, BMI, waist circumference, gender, cardiometabolic attributes. The randomization process is designed to balance the groups across key variables, and the results reported in Table 1 supported this – no significant group differences were observed between the three experimental groups for all 31 characteristics.

Q7 Which relationships were reported to be statistically significant (or not)?

The results compared the effects of the interventions on various health outcomes, and the differences between groups across various markers of cardiac risk. For instance, comparisons between the green MED, MED, and HDG groups showed significant differences in terms of decline in weight loss after 6 months:

> The green MED (–6.2 ± 5.9 kg) and MED (–5.4 ± 5.6 kg) group participants... exhibited similar weight loss that was greater than in the HDG group (–1.5 ± 3.9 kg, $p < 0.001$ for both comparisons) [3].

Secondarily, the Framingham Risk score decreased as well.

> ...the 10-year Framingham Risk score significantly decreased in all study groups (HDG 13.3% to 11.2%, $p = 0.001$; MED 11.5% to 9.5%, $p < 0.001$; green MED 13.7% to 10.4%, $p < 0.001$) [3].

Q8 How strong were the relationships?

Table 3 in the article shows changes in metabolic markers and cardiovascular risk within and between experimental groups. Of the three experimental groups, the green MED group showed the greatest reduction across most metabolic markers and risk measures, differing most significantly from the HDG group.

For instance, the study assessed the effect of each intervention on weight loss, measured in kilograms. Participants in all experimental groups, on average, lost weight – on average, the HDG group lost 1.5 kg, the MED group lost 5.4 kg, and the green MED group lost 6.2 kg. Similarly, reduction in waist circumference was significantly greater in the green MED intervention group – 8.6 cm – than the other two groups.

Findings also show a reduction in cardiovascular risk, as measured by the Framingham Risk score. The greatest risk reduction also occurred among the green MED intervention group, although the difference risk scores between the MED and green MED groups were not significant.

BOX 9.1   ABSOLUTE AND RELATIVE MEASURES OF EFFECT

Measures such as weight and waist circumference are easily understood measures of impact or effect in a particular population. Many studies use these *absolute* measures of the effect. In contrast, *relative* measures of effect are more complex and are understood comparatively – the comparative impact of, say, exposure to a breastfeeding program versus non-exposure. The use of a relative or absolute measure of effect depends on the study's aim.

Reading the discussion

Q9 What were the strengths and limitations of the study?

As an experiment that randomly assigns subjects to experimental groups, covariates are evenly distributed and, hence, their potentially confounding effects on outcomes would be limited. This enhances confidence that the change in cardiometabolic outcomes resulted from the interventions.

Certain study limitations were identified, however. The study sample included a disproportionate number of men (just 35 women, 259 men). This might limit the ability to apply these results to women. The study also relied on self-reports of dietary compliance and physical outside the lunchroom setting. Further, the study assessed change over a six-month period, so the effects of diets over the longer term were not assessed.

Finally, the strength of the study is also a key limitation. Lunches were monitored and distributed, certain items for the MED or green MED meals were prescribed, and calories were restricted. The controlled conditions enabled researchers to isolate the effects of the interventions on weight loss, waist circumference, and other outcomes. This strengthens the ability interpret the association as a causal one. Nonetheless, the controlled conditions of the dietary intervention would be difficult to replicate in natural, real-world settings. Thus, the study mainly contributes to our scientific understanding of how dietary ingredients might influence cardiometabolic risk more than it does a practical understanding of how to foster the everyday consumption of these ingredients.

Q10 What were the implications of the study for research and practice?

Health practitioners seldom base practice decisions on the results of a single primary study, however compelling these results might be. In the case of MED diets, results have been consistent with other, similar studies that point to the cardiometabolic benefits of a diet rich in plants and proteins and light on red meats. Although replicating the study outside a controlled context might be challenging, the study's evidence lends further support to the body of evidence on the effects of diet on cardiovascular health. The evidence can inform those at risk for obesity or metabolic disorders to incorporate food items with nutritional content similar to those in Mediterranean and green Mediterranean diets.

Recap

This chapter provided examples of analytically reading peer-reviewed experimental studies that use natural-, quasi-, and true experimental designs. The chapter uses the ten analytical questions to activate the reading process and guide readers in a critical examination of each study's methodology, results, and implications.

The examples included: (1) a natural experiment that examines the effects of minimum wage legislation on depression, (2) a quasi-experiment that tests the effects of a breastfeeding education program on breastfeeding duration and exclusiveness, and (3) the effects of the Mediterranean diet programs on cardiometabolic risk.

Each example illustrated how the analytical questions can be used to examine a study and assess its practical implications. The example's aim is to enhance the ability to identify and critically assess the strengths and limitations of observational studies to facilitate a deeper understanding of the implications of experimental research for evidence-based practice.

References

1. Reeves A, McKee M, Mackenbach J, Whitehead M, Stuckler D. Introduction of a national minimum wage reduced depressive symptoms in low-wage workers: A quasi-natural experiment in the UK. *Health Econ.* 2017;26(5):639–655. doi:10.1002/hec.3336.
2. van Dellen SA, Wisse B, Mobach MP, Dijkstra A. The effect of a breastfeeding support programme on breastfeeding duration and exclusivity: A quasi-experiment. *BMC Public Health.* 2019;19:993. doi:10.1186/s12889-019-7331-y.
3. Tsaban G, Meir AY, Rinott E, Zelicha H, Kaplan A, Shalev A, et al. The effect of green Mediterranean diet on cardiometabolic risk; A randomised controlled trial. *Heart.* 2021;107(13):1054–1061. doi:10.1136/heartjnl-2020-317802.

10

QUALITATIVE RESEARCH DESIGNS

Overview of qualitative designs

Qualitative health research is an interpretative science that developed out of the social sciences rather than from the observational and experimental sciences. In contrast to quantitative research, which aims to predict and control outcomes, qualitative research aims to generate insights and understanding of human experiences and the diverse perspectives of various human groups.

Aims of qualitative studies

Qualitative studies in health science aim to improve our understanding of experiences and perspectives of health and illness, of patients, clients, caregivers, and caregiving. Here are some examples of study aims as stated in qualitative research articles.

1 "to explore the subjective experiences of diagnosis, treatment processes and meaning of recovery in children and adolescents suffering from OCD and provide a conceptual model of the illness" [1]
2 "to explore diet-related intra-couple dynamics and to reconstruct dietary concepts and associated influencing factors among older couples" [2]
3 "to understand users' perspectives regarding a mobile social networking intervention to promote physical activity" [3]
4 "to explore how female college students use of Instagram, and if using Instagram impacts body image" [4]
5 "to investigate how patients with OA [osteoarthritis] experience their disease and care process, highlighting potential elements that can enhance or spoil it, to optimize the quality of care" [5]

The open-ended nature of these research aims is evident, focusing mainly on understanding human experiences and perspectives. The exploration is often open-ended, conducted

DOI: 10.4324/9781003595663-12

with few expectations about what the results will be. Qualitative studies do not test hypotheses, but are often used, instead, to generate further questions and hypotheses while also advancing our understanding of the experiences of others and ourselves.

Qualitative research aims to present findings that are credible and trustworthy in capturing the experiences and perspectives of patients, clients, caregiving, and caregivers with respect to health, illness, and health care. Credibility has to do with how plausible the findings and interpretations are and how accurately they capture participants' experiences and perspectives. Trustworthiness pertains to the transparency of the methods used to generate the findings, enabling the study to be replicated, confirmed, and transferred to other contexts. Trustworthy results are also credible. Qualitative studies are assessed in terms of the credibility and trustworthiness of their findings.

Questions for analytically reading qualitative studies

We propose ten questions for analyzing qualitative studies. The first two and last two of the 10 questions identified for analyzing qualitative studies are the same as those used for analyzing quantitative studies. The first two ask about the study's relevance and design. The last two ask about the contributions, limitations, and implications of the study.

Questions pertaining to qualitative methods and results differ substantially, however. This difference is mainly due to the collection and analysis of non-numeric data that characterizes qualitative research. We identify distinct analytical questions to be considered by readers to critically assess the methods and results of such studies.

The credibility and trustworthiness of qualitative findings depend on the methods employed to collect and analyze non-numeric data. We propose three questions to ask the Methods section of qualitative research articles:

Q3 How and why were subjects selected?
Q4 What data were collected, and how?
Q5 What analytical strategies were used to limit biases and enhance the study's credibility?

Likewise, the results of qualitative research mainly take the form of themes and theories that cut across and capture the data that was collected. The credibility and trustworthiness of these findings, however, depends on the quality of the methods used to generate them. We propose three questions to ask the Results section of qualitative research articles.

Q6 How were the sample and setting characterized?
Q7 Was enough data presented to support emergent themes and theories?
Q8 How credible were the themes and theories that emerged from the data?

Each question is discussed below, and examples are presented in Chapter 11.

Q3 How and why were subjects selected?

This question is asked to help gauge how transferable the results are to other settings and populations – where and to whom the findings might apply. Qualitative studies often include a much smaller number of cases than is characteristic of quantitative studies. Qualitative studies often sacrifice breadth of the findings for depth and novelty of their insights. As is often the case in primary research more generally, however, selecting participants is based on practical convenience, having to rely on accessible volunteers. Volunteers may have different experiences or stronger voices than less accessible, non-volunteers. Critical readers will surely consider this when assessing similarity to other settings or people.

Other qualitative studies sample purposively, deliberately selecting certain settings and cases to achieve specific study aims. For instance, studies might seek to maximize variation in sampling to capture a wide range of perspectives. Criterion sampling involves selecting cases that meet pre-defined criteria, often to ensure that a range of views are expressed – e.g., perspectives from people of different socioeconomic status, geographic location, or racial backgrounds. Extreme or deviant case sampling is used to highlight variation among cases, to emphasize processes obscured under average conditions or by typical cases. Snowball sampling may be used to identify rare or hard to find cases, by leveraging networks of initial participants to locate and recruit others.

The nature of sampling – convenience or purposive – will depend on the aim of the study. Whether out of practical convenience or for a specific purpose, understanding the nature of the study sample is important for understanding the transferability of qualitative findings – where and to whom the qualitative results might apply. Transferability may be assessed based on the support the evidence shows to a more general theory or how closely the attributes of the sampled cases resemble those of the group or cases the reader is targeting.

Q4   What data were collected, and how?

Qualitative data are non-numeric and collected from various sources – e.g., field observations, documents, online posts, and interview responses. They also come as photographs, images, or cultural artifacts that researchers analyze and interpret. For instance, the photovoice qualitative approach uses photos from study participants to express and reflect their perspectives on life experiences [6]. Some qualitative studies collect and compile non-numeric data from multiple sources or combine it with numeric data in a case study (see Box 10.1 and Example 11.2).

BOX 10.1   CASE STUDIES

Case studies are a kind of qualitative, descriptive study that investigates, in detail, a specific case or bounded system (e.g., an organization, group, community, or individual). For instance, the case might be a village in upper Egypt, a unique primary care medical practice, or an Olympic swimmer. Researchers will describe these cases in detail to generate and illustrate ideas for training student-practitioners, or to gain insight into an unusual or instructive case. The very detailed findings highlight the unique qualities of the case, which makes it challenging to directly apply findings to other cases that differ in important ways.

Most commonly, however, qualitative data are transcripts from in-depth interviews or focus groups. The interview process usually involves the development of an interview guide that includes unstructured open-ended questions or semi-structured questions to foster consistency and assure comprehensive coverage of relevant items. To gain insight into the experiences and perspectives of research subjects, interviews may take an hour or more to generate dozens of pages of transcripts to be analyzed.

Skill in interviewing is essential to build trust with respondents. Otherwise, responses are likely to be brief, superficial, or aimed at maintaining social approval rather than providing a true reflection of their experiences or perspectives. While the interview process poses a risk of researcher and response biases (Appendix B), the credibility of qualitative interviewing is enhanced with trained and experienced interviewers.

Based on the sample and data collected, readers can begin to consider how thick or thin the data promises to be. Qualitative researchers sometimes refer to data collected until "saturation" is reached – the point where additional data contribute little more in terms of insight and understanding. The more data that is collected, the more credible the findings tend to be.

Q5   *What analytical strategies were used to limit biases and enhance the study's credibility?*

A major challenge for qualitative analysis is that text passages, images, and other non-numeric data can mean different things to different people, and no single interpretation is necessarily the true and accurate one. Further, subjects' responses will vary and reflect their unique experiences and perspectives. Thus, qualitative studies not only require that enough data are collected to construct a credible set of findings, but they also require a systematic approach to analyzing this data to guard against various biases that can undermine this credibility.

Unlike quantitative research where agreed-upon procedures are used to statistically analyze numeric data, qualitative research must take distinctly different measures to reduce the risk of bias and to enhance the credibility of the findings. Though the analytical processes for qualitative studies vary in their details, Figure 10.1 shows the process of transforming raw text data into meaningful themes and theories.

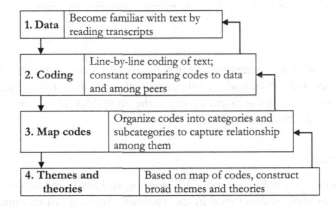

FIGURE 10.1   Coding and analyzing qualitative data.

First, researchers will familiarize themselves with the data by reading several or all the transcripts and develop an agreed-to set of rules for attaching meaningful codes to the words and passages of the transcripts. Using these rules, one or more researchers will engage in line-by-line coding of the text. Codes will be organized into categories and subcategories that should fit together logically or that represent components of a larger theory. From mapping of codes, themes or theories are constructed to capture the experiences or perspectives expressed in the data.

Coding non-numeric data to eventually translate codes to themes is a basic strategy found in virtually every qualitative study. The themes emerge from an iterative process, where codes and categories are initially fluid but gradually solidify as researchers discuss and gain consensus on the overarching themes.

Analyst triangulation

Reaching consensus among diverse researchers is a fundamental component of the qualitative analysis process. The biases of one researcher can serve as a check on those of other researchers. This check is enhanced where researchers come from different disciplines, institutions, or professions. The reliance on consensus in developing codes and themes is referred to as "analyst triangulation" (see Box 10.2).

BOX 10.2 ANALYST TRIANGULATION VERSUS SINGLE CODERS

Often two or three members of the research team will review a subset of interviews, develop an agreed-upon coding scheme, and independently code the data. Codes can then be compared, and reliability of coding can be checked. There are some advantages to having just one member of the team engaging in coding, however. Coding is less costly and more consistent with a single coder. Further, single coders often have special expertise in the subject matter and, therefore, are often best suited to understanding subtleties and meanings of the text. Finally, another common form of analyst triangulation is to have two or more members of the team independently code a sample of the data, develop an agreed-upon coding scheme, and, have one member code the remaining data.

Reflexive practice

A second analytic strategy is engagement in reflexive practice during the process of coding and the transformation of codes to themes. In this practice, researchers deliberately reflect on how their own biases might influence the analytic process. Identifying biases is the first step toward limiting their effects.

Negative case analysis

Negative case analysis involves intentionally seeking and analyzing cases that are inconsistent with major themes developed in the analysis. An in-depth examination of how negative or contrary cases differ from other cases can sharpen and help define the limits of the analysis, while also guarding against confirmation bias.

Other strategies in qualitative analysis

Member checking, peer debriefing, and maintaining an audit trail may be used to enhance the transparency and credibility of the study by fostering external review of the research process and results. Member checking involves seeking corrective feedback from participants to ensure the accuracy of data and interpretation. Peer debriefing involves seeking corrective feedback from expert peers on the methods and the interpretation of the results. An audit trail is the ongoing record of the data collection, coding, and interpretation processes that others can scrutinize and possibly replicate.

In the analysis subsection, readers may find several of these strategies outlined and used to enhance the credibility of qualitative studies. It is often not feasible to engage many of these strategies to limit bias, and this may compromise the credibility of the findings [7].

Q6   *How were the sample and setting characterized?*

The first table will usually characterize the results of the sampling process. For interview studies, this table usually describes attributes of sampled participants – e.g., age, sex, race, education, and health status. The results may also describe the setting – e.g., attributes of the community, size and type of organization or clinical practice from which participants are drawn. This adds context and richness to the data and helps inform the transferability of the results.

The table and surrounding text will describe the nature of the sample and setting – the size and diversity. Analytical readers will ask where and to whom this data might apply and not apply.

Q7   *Was enough data presented to support emergent themes and theories?*

Results of qualitative studies are often represented by direct quotes from the participants that reflect their experiences and perspectives. Multiple quotes, observations, or other anecdotes are used to describe the setting along with participants' experiences and views. The richer the description, the more credible the study's broader narrative tends to be. Readers should be satisfied with the thoroughness and believability of the account.

Q8   *How credible were the themes and theories that emerged from the data?*

Coding text data and generating themes and theories is an interpretative process that aims to construct and convey a credible description of the experiences and perspectives of research subjects. The credibility of the resulting themes or theories rests on the richness of the data and tools used to limit bias in the analysis and interpretation of the data. Thus, analytical readers will ask whether the themes, subthemes, and theories reported are coherent, plausible, and credible. In so doing, they may also ask where their own biases lie when making that assessment.

Trustworthiness of qualitative research

Readers will first gauge whether the account is credible – does the researcher's account accurately reflect participants' realities? This involves not only describing what themes were reported but also critically analyzing the process of data collection and analysis used to identify them. Theories and themes that credibly capture the experiences, meanings, and perspectives of cases are also assessed in terms of their trustworthiness. Trustworthiness pertains to the credibility and transferability of findings to other people or settings.

In qualitative research, transferability does not involve generalizing findings through statistical inference. Transferability in qualitative studies has to do with how well findings apply to other groups, individuals, or settings. This often depends on the resemblance of the study population to individuals or groups the reader is concerned with. For instance, indicators of resemblance might be age, gender, socioeconomic status, race/ethnicity, or religion. Transferability may also occur analytically, as well, where findings of the study support a general theory which, in turn, applies to other people and settings.

Strengths and limitations of qualitative studies

A major strength of qualitative studies is the construction of a detailed, complex, and insightful account of human experiences and perspectives as expressed by the research participants. The experiences and perspectives are lodged within a particular social context as well and this may become part of the study's broader, holistic account. Accurately reflecting the experiences and perspectives fosters greater understanding which, in turn, leads to more productive engagements among professionals, clients, and others more generally.

Since qualitative research involves interpreting non-numeric data, it also faces potential subjective and research biases that may affect the findings and interpretation. There are several tools available to identify and limit these biases, though for various reasons they are not consistently employed in qualitative studies [7].

Since qualitative research provides detailed accounts of particular individuals in particular settings, it also faces the challenge of "transferability" – i.e., applying results from one group and setting to others. Samples in qualitative studies may bear little resemblance to groups and settings of interest. While theoretically meaningful, transferring results to other settings should be done with caution and care.

Recap

This chapter described the essential components of a qualitative approach to health research. The approach is rooted in interpretive social science and aims to deepen our understanding of the diverse meanings, experiences, and perspectives of health, illness, and caregiving. Unlike quantitative research, which collects *numeric* data for statistical analysis, qualitative research collects and analyzes *non-numeric* data. Rather than aiming to predict and control health outcomes, qualitative research aims to capture and communicate the diverse experiences, meanings, and perspectives of health and healthcare. To enhance the credibility and trustworthiness of qualitative accounts, the chapter described various strategies for collecting and analyzing qualitative data that are designed to limit sources of research biases.

Finally, the chapter introduced questions designed to guide and activate readers in the critical analysis of qualitative studies. The questions that pertain to the methods and results of qualitative studies differ from those relevant to quantitative studies. Nonetheless, the questions serve the same purpose – to activate the reading process and foster a critical analysis of how findings from qualitative studies and their contribution to our understanding of the meanings, experiences, and perspectives of health and illness.

References

1. Sravanti L, Kommu JVS, Girimaji SC, Seshadri S. Lived experiences of children and adolescents with obsessive–compulsive disorder: Interpretative phenomenological analysis. *Child Adolesc Psychiatry Ment Health*. 2022;16(1):44. doi:10.1186/s13034-022-00478-7.
2. Wirsching D, Baer NR, Anton V, Schenk L. Dietary concepts in the dyad: Results from a qualitative study of middle-aged and older couples. *Appetite*. 2022;175:106020. doi:10.1016/j.appet.2022.106020.
3. Tong L, Coiera E, Laranjo L. Using a mobile social networking app to promote physical activity: A qualitative study of users' perspectives. *J Med Internet Res*. 2018;20(12):e11439. doi:10.2196/11439.
4. Baker N, Ferszt G, Breines JG. A qualitative study exploring female college students' Instagram use and body image. *Cyberpsychol Behav Soc Netw*. 2019;22(4):277–282. doi:10.1089/cyber.2018.0420.
5. Battista S, Manoni M, Dell'Isola A, Englund M, Palese A, Testa M. Giving an account of patients' experience: A qualitative study on the care process of hip and knee osteoarthritis. *Health Expect*. 2022;25(3):1140–1156. doi:10.1111/hex.13468.
6. Im D, Pyo J, Lee H, Jung H, Ock M. Qualitative research in healthcare: Data analysis. *J Prev Med Public Health*. 2023;56(2):100–110. doi:10.3961/jpmph.22.471.
7. Raskind IG, Shelton RC, Comeau DL, Cooper HLF, Griffith DM, Kegler MC. A review of qualitative data analysis practices in health education and health behavior research. *Health Educ Behav*. 2019;46(1):32–39. doi:10.1177/1090198118795019.

11

ANALYTICALLY READING QUALITATIVE STUDIES

This Chapter provides two examples to illustrate the process of analytically reading peer-reviewed qualitative studies. The examples use ten analytical questions for qualitative studies. As discussed previously, the first and last two questions – on relevance, design, limitations, and implications – are identical to those used to examine quantitative studies (and the review studies described in Chapter 13). Q3–Q5 and Q6–Q8 are used to analyze the methods and results of qualitative studies (Table 11.1).

Example 11.2 illustrates a mixed-methods approach that uses both quantitative and qualitative study designs. Often, the results of qualitative and quantitative arms of a mixed-methods study are reported in separate articles, and this is the case in this example.

Example 11.1 illustrates a straightforward qualitative interview study that aimed to explore perceptions of musculoskeletal pain and how these perceptions were accommodated in clinical decisions. The results of the study reinforced a fundamental principle

TABLE 11.1 Ten (10) questions for analytically reading qualitative studies

Section	Question
Title, Abstract, Introduction	Q1 Is the study relevant?
	Q2 What was the study design?
Methods	Q3 How and why were subjects selected?
	Q4 What data were collected, and how?
	Q5 What analytical strategies were used to limit biases and enhance the study's credibility?
Results	Q6 How were the sample and setting characterized?
	Q7 Was enough data presented to support emergent themes and theories?
	Q8 How credible were the themes and theories that emerged from the data?
Discussion and Conclusion	Q9 What were the strengths and limitations of the study?
	Q10 What were the implications of the study for research and practice?

DOI: 10.4324/9781003595663-13

of EBP highlighting the importance of client engagement, as captured in the title: "A preference for dialogue".

Example 11.1   Analytically reading a qualitative study

Title: "A preference for dialogue: exploring the influence of patient preferences on clinical decision making and treatment in primary care physiotherapy". [1]

Inspectional reading

The article title provides a picture of the health topic – how patients' preferences affect clinical decision making in primary care physiotherapy (PT). From the abstract, readers learn that the study explores involvement in decision making for patients experiencing musculoskeletal pain. According to the Introduction section, there are few studies on the topic, even though the problem is common in PT. The introduction suggests that better understanding of patients' preferences will facilitate evidence-based practice.

A qualitative study design was used to explore the topic. While its relevance for physiotherapists seems clear, the evidence could also be applicable for other healthcare practitioners who seek to foster patient engagement and evidence-based practice.

Reading the methods

Q3 How and why were subjects selected?

Participants were patients in physiotherapy for treatment of musculoskeletal pain. The setting was one of an urban outpatient physiotherapy clinic with a "mixed socio-economic profile that serves patients of all ages". The clinic was located in Sweden. Included were patients who recently experienced physiotherapy treatment and who spoke and understood Swedish.

Participants were purposively selected "to maximize variation by gender, age and pain location". As is sometimes the case, the first table is shown the Methods section, providing a brief description of the participants. These included nine men and nine women, aged 23 and 77 years of age, with diverse professional and educational backgrounds. Pain location also varied: back ($n = 6$), neck ($n = 5$), shoulder ($n = 4$), and neck/shoulder ($n = 3$). Thus, the sample showed variation in the circumstances of subjects, and, presumably, a variety of perspectives.

Q4 What data were collected, and how?

Data were collected from individual interviews – nine were conducted in person, nine were conducted by phone. One researcher conducted all 18 interviews. This adds consistency of the data collection process. The interview guide (provided in a supplemental table) featured several open-ended questions to enable participants to elaborate in their responses. Interviews averaged 22 minutes and ranged from 15 to 42 minutes. Interviews were audio-recorded and transcribed in preparation for the analysis.

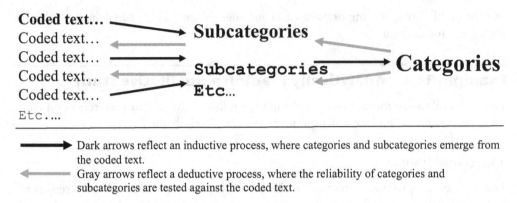

Dark arrows reflect an inductive process, where categories and subcategories emerge from the coded text.

Gray arrows reflect a deductive process, where the reliability of categories and subcategories are tested against the coded text.

FIGURE 11.1   The iterative process characteristic of qualitative research for analyzing coded text.

Q5 What analytical strategies were used to limit biases and enhance the study's credibility?

A qualitative "content analysis" was conducted where transcripts were read several times to gain a detailed understanding of the text and the preferences surrounding clinical decision making. The coding protocol involved the independent coding of three transcripts by two researchers (analyst triangulation) to cross-check and verify the codes to be used for coding all of the transcripts ($n = 18$).

Once the coding process was complete, the coded text was sorted into subcategories and categories in an iterative process to characterize the content of the transcripts (Figure 11.1).

As is common in qualitative research, categories and subcategories are seen to come from *inductive* reasoning where categories emerge from a detailed examination of the coded text. The dark arrows in the figure represent this inductive process. In contrast, the gray arrows represent the *deductive* side of this process. Deductive reasoning involves assessing the credibility of the abstract categories be testing them against coded text.

The back-and-forth between categories and coded text reflects what is the *iterative* nature of qualitative analysis. Categories and subcategories tend to be fluid early in the qualitative analysis, but firm up as they become checked and rechecked when new data come in and as discussions with the research team evolve.

The Results section describes the results of this iterative process.

Reading the results

Q6 How were the sample and setting characterized?

Table 1 in the study provides demographic and health information about the sample. The sample aimed to maximize variation in the sample. Respondents varied substantially with respect to gender, age, profession, education, pain location and symptom duration. All respondents appear to have had at least some undergraduate training, and several had graduate training.

Q7 Was enough data presented to support emergent themes and theories?

Readers will find a description of the themes that emerged from the transcripts. First, the article identified four broad categories and 14 subcategories that emerged from the coding and analysis of the transcripts. The article described each category and subcategory and used one to three quotes to illustrate their content using the voices of patient-respondents. For instance, content of the subcategory labeled "A good listener" was supported by this patient quote

> I think she listened really well, actually. Definitely. And that's… that's a big problem with this type of pain/…/She showed a very big understanding for it, and didn't just dismiss it. Instead she said that… she admitted that there was a problem there [1].

The content of this subcategory others, fell under the larger category labeled as "Two-way communication". With this category, three other categories surfaced to describe the content of the transcripts: "My views matter, "Leaving decisions to the physio" and "Physiotherapy influences preferences". Cutting across all four categories was a single theme labeled as: "A preference for dialogue – communication essential for collaborative rehabilitation".

The narrative provided in the Results describes the four categories, and 14 subcategories, using quotations from patient-respondents to illustrate. Were these categories sufficiently grounded in the data to offer a rich and credible representation of patients' perspectives?

Q8 How credible were the themes and theories that emerged from the data?

In this example, from 18 transcripts researchers identified 14 subcategories that fall under 4 themes. These 4 themes point toward a single, overarching theme: "a preference for dialogue". Analytic readers will ask whether categories and subcategories logically connect, along with the strength of the evidence supporting PT patients' overall preference for dialogue.

Reading the discussion

Q9 What were the strengths and limitations of the study?

The article discussed correspondence of the study findings with findings from other qualitative investigations of patients under orthopedic and primary care. Other studies illustrate patients' preferences for being informed, even if they leave the decision to the practitioner.

The question of how trustworthy a study's findings persist in qualitative research. Trustworthiness is largely based on the credibility and transferability of study findings. In this case, credibility of the research is strengthened by variation in the sample to represent a variety of perspectives, by analyst triangulation in the coding process, and using quotations to illustrate the various categories and subcategories. A structured interview process fostered consistency across interviews, reducing researcher bias.

Other analytical strategies were not used – peer debriefing, member checking, and negative case analysis. The study risks the effects of biases associated with the interviewer's potential influence on responses, as well as the respondents' potential desire to respond in socially approved ways.

The findings are drawn from patients of a PT practice in Sweden. This may limit the transferability of these results to other settings. First, Swedish physiotherapists enjoy sufficient autonomy to enable therapists and patients to engage in dialogue regarding decisions and care. This autonomy is not enjoyed by physiotherapists everywhere. Second, Swedish patients may well be different from patients elsewhere regarding preferences, their eagerness to engage with the therapist, or their inclination to defer to the therapist. This also complicates the transferability of the results to different populations and settings.

Q10 *What were the implications of the study for research and practice?*

Seldom do results from a single study have much of an effect on decisions or practice. It is usually when evidence from several studies accumulates that professional practice will change. The article suggests that dialogue with clients may be most important for problems such as pain management where diverse options are available (e.g., acupuncture, massage) and no single option is clearly superior to others. In addition, the assessment that clients maintain a "preference for dialogue" upholds ethical principles of individual and patient autonomy and reinforces practice that is evidence based.

Example 11.2   Mixing qualitative and quantitative designs

Title: "Beyond the pain: A qualitative study exploring the physical therapy experience in patients with chronic low back pain". [2]

Studies that combine quantitative and qualitative approaches are referred to as "mixed-methods" studies. The mixing of quantitative and qualitative methods may proceed in different sequences. For instance, a study took a quantitative approach in randomly selecting of 5000 "tweets" about cannabis edibles and a qualitative approach to coding the tweets and identifying themes about their meaning. [3] Other studies may use qualitative methods and open-ended interviews to gain an insight into respondents' perspectives, but also to inform a structured questionnaire sent to a broader population followed by a statistical analysis of the responses.

Often, however, qualitative and quantitative approaches are used concurrently by combining randomized control trials (RCTs) with qualitative interviews. For instance, researchers might wish to assess the alignment of the "objective" effects of an intervention with the "perceived" effects of the intervention among participants. This mixed-methods approach can also aid in adjusting interventions in ways to make them more acceptable to clients.

Example 11.2 illustrates a mixed-methods approach that aims to explore PT patients' experiences with an intervention designed to reduce chronic low back pain. The qualitative study of patients' experiences is embedded within an RCT.

Inspectional reading

The title and abstract indicate that a "mixed-methods" approach was used – a qualitative approach together with a randomized control trial (RCT) aimed to describe the experience of PT among a mainly low-income minority population with chronic low back pain (cLBP). The RCT phase of the study compared the effects of yoga, PT, and educational interventions. The effects of the interventions are described in a separate article [4]. "Beyond the Pain" focuses on the qualitative phase of the study.

Reading the methods

Q3 How and why were subjects selected?

Subjects were drawn from those who completed the 12-week phase of the "parent" RCT. Invitations to participate were sent to 102 participants in the RCT, and twelve (12) agreed to be interviewed. Although response rates this low response are not unusual, it does suggest the potential for volunteer bias, where findings will reflect the perceptions of the most eager and satisfied study participants. It difficult to gauge how well the perceptions reflect the views of 102 participants in the RCT.

Q4 How and what data were data collected?

Data were collected by semi-structured interviews. Interviews lasted between 30 and 60 minutes, using a version of an interview guide adapted from another study. Open-ended questions with follow-up probative questions enabled participants to provide open, detailed responses about their experiences with PT care.

An interview guide was used to standardize the interview process, and to ensure the various dimensions of a topic are covered in every interview. The guide identified several questions, along with several prompts designed to expand the dialogue around participants' satisfaction with the PT intervention. For instance,

- "What was your initial experience like with physical therapy?"
- "How has physical therapy influenced how you feel about LBP [low back pain]? How you cope with it?"
- "Thinking about what you got out of your physical experience, which is more important to you – mental effects… or pain relief? Why?"
- "How has your perception of physical therapy changed over the course of this study?" [2]

Interviews were audio-recorded and transcribed. The transcribed interviews provide the primary, non-numeric data to be qualitatively analyzed. Some data from the RCT phase was pulled and used to compare with and complement the qualitative data.

Q5 What analytical strategies were used to limit biases and enhance the study's credibility?

Transcripts were independently coded by two researchers and disagreements were resolved by a third researcher (analyst triangulation). The six-member team was multi-disciplinary, consisting of clinicians from 3 health professions and a medical anthropologist. Thus, diverse perspectives were available to analyze and interpret the text. The team engaged in reflection throughout the process: "We continued to discuss reflexivity throughout the analysis and attempted to interpret and report the meanings and words of the participants as they were intended".

The study also presented data that were "contrary to our narrative", an analytic strategy designed to limit confirmation bias and over-generalization, thereby more clearly delimiting the major findings.

The team was able to assess whether respondents' accounts aligned with quantitative data from the RCT. This "triangulation of methods" is available to mixed-methods studies. The study blinded researchers to these findings so as not to bias the interpretations – knowing the quantitative findings might skew qualitative coding toward alignment with these findings. Hence, findings were withheld from the researchers until after qualitative analysis was completed (a form of "blinding").

Reading the results

Q6 How were the sample and setting characterized?

As discussed, the study relied on volunteer participants. Participants consisted of 12 individuals, mostly female (92%), mostly black (75%), and of middle age (mean=51.9 years). Gross income for all participants was below $40,000/year. According to the quantitative findings of the RCT, all participants were experiencing high levels of pain and disability at baseline. Further, pain scores decreased for all 12 participants in the PT arm, and disability scores decreased for 10 of the 12. In short, all or most study participants experienced improvement in pain and disability scores. In regard to the success of the treatments after 12 weeks, it is unclear how well the study sample represented other participants in the parent RCT.

Q7 Was enough data presented to support emergent themes and theories?

Based largely on the frequency of codes, three distinct themes were developed: (1) empowerment through education and exercise; (2) interconnectedness; and 3) improvements in pain, body mechanics, and mood. Underneath each theme were several subthemes that were supported by several more coded passages (see Table 11.2).

Themes were described in the Results and were supported by several quotes from the participants. For instance, the *mastery of experience* subtheme received support from an African American woman participant who was encouraged to take an active approach to managing her cLBP

> Instead of just taking medication or putting a hot pack on… it felt good, you know, I'm taking charge of healing myself, controlling myself [2].

TABLE 11.2 From subthemes to themes in qualitative research

Subtheme	Theme
Mastery of experience	Empowerment through education and exercise
Verbal persuasion	
Vicarious experience	
Physiological state	
Patient-therapist relationship	Interconnectedness
Patient-patient relationship	
Negative patient-therapist relationship	
Improved mood	Improvements in pain, body mechanics and
Decreased pain	mood
Increased flexibility	
Improved strength/posture	
No change in pain	

Adapted from "The experience of physical therapy in underserved participants withchronic low back pain". Subthemes and themes from [2]

The quote appears logically connected to the larger subtheme – reference to "taking charge of healing myself" aligns with the subtheme "mastery of experience. Additionally, this subtheme logically connects with the larger theme about empowerment through education and exercise.

The richness and coherence of qualitative data as it relates to codes, subthemes, and themes underlies the overall credibility of the findings.

Q8 *How credible were the themes and theories that emerged from the data?*

The study used several analytical tools to guard against research bias. The study engaged in analyst triangulation and triangulation of methods. Analyst triangulation requires that multiple team members are engaged in coding and the development of themes. The team was represented by diverse health professionals who likely brought different perspectives to the process. Bringing them together to code and develop themes broadens the perspectives and diminishes the chance of research bias. This enhances the credibility of the themes and subthemes developed.

Triangulation of methods involves analyzing a single phenomenon using different research approaches. In this case, qualitative results regarding improved pain, mood, and body mechanics largely correspond with quantitative findings showing experiencing less pain and disability.

The correspondence between quantitative and qualitative findings strengthens their overall credibility. In addition, the study took steps to blind the coders from the results of the quantitative study until all the interviews were analyzed. This protects against researcher (specifically, interpreter) bias, and enhances the credibility of the findings.

Reading the discussion

Q9 *What were the strengths and limitations of the study?*

Reflective practice, analyst triangulation, triangulation of methods (with blinding) contributes to the credibility of the results. Although the study suggests an examination of cases contrary to their narrative, there is limited discussion of these cases. Also, the themes constructed were not shared with respondents or outside experts for feedback – member checking and peer debriefing. Though desirable, member checking and peer debriefing is more often not feasible.

Importantly, the analysis and results are consistent with evidence from other studies that affirm the importance of developing a therapeutic alliance with patients. The Discussion elaborates on the theme of empowerment, connecting four subthemes to Bandura's theory of self-efficacy. Self-efficacy is a precursor to empowerment. Results that are consistent with Bandura's theory may be transferable to other contexts as well (see Box 11.1).

The data are based on a convenience sample of 12 participants in a larger RCT, and 11 of the 12 were female patients. This leaves open the question of how transferable the findings are to male patients. As important, however, is the response rate – 12 of 102 patients in the intervention phase agreed to participate. The 12 who participated expressed satisfaction with the program, and almost all showed a reduction in pain and disability. In contrast, it is entirely plausible that the 90 who did not participate were, on average, less satisfied and would have expressed views that the study could not capture. The Discussion suggests that additional interviews of non-responders, particularly those reporting less favorable outcomes, would be called for to enhance transferability of the results.

BOX 11.1   ANALYTIC GENERALIZATION AND TRANSFERABILITY [5]

Health professionals are keenly interested in transferring findings to specific cases. They may assess how cases in a study sample resemble the specific cases of interest. For instance, a set of cases may be similar in age, gender, ethnicity, education. But professionals might also assess study findings that support a theory which has general application to various settings and people--analytic generalization. Professionals should take care not to over-generalize findings based on their resemblance to specific cases or their support for a general theory. As discussed in Chapter 15, professionals must consider the unique qualities of specific cases before transferring or applying study findings.

Q10   What were the implications of the study for research and practice?

Although the sample itself was limited, study findings do support the benefits of empowering patients – patient self-efficacy and empowerment seem to coincide with improvements in outcomes and well-being. Understanding the role of self-efficacy and empowerment in the care of often disempowered populations may be particularly salient for other practices.

The Discussion also refers the historic mistreatment of African American patients by health professionals, and the corresponding distrust that often produces. Thus, evidence of the beneficial effects of building a solid therapeutic relationship that fosters patients' self-efficacy in this often underserved and understudied population may resonate more widely among health professionals.

Recap

This Chapter presented two examples to illustrate analytically reading peer-reviewed qualitative studies. The Chapter used the ten analytical questions to activate the reading process and guide readers in a critical examination of each study's methods, results, and implications.

The first example showed how patients' preferences influenced physiotherapy treatments for musculoskeletal pain, highlighting the importance of dialogue in clinical settings. The example illustrated common strategies for data collection (e.g., purposive sampling and in-depth interviews) and data analysis (e.g., analyst triangulation). This qualitative interview study underscored the principle of client engagement in evidence-based practice (EBP), reflecting the necessity of patient-centered care in physiotherapy. The second example showed the qualitative portion of a mixed-methods study designed to capture patients' perspectives of the treatment intervention used in an RCT. The results of the RCT were reported separately, but the study showed an alignment between positive effects and respondents' positive experiences.

This mixed-methods approach provided a more complete view of the effects of the treatment intervention and its effects.

Each example illustrated the application of analytical questions to assess a study's relevance, design, data collection and analysis methods, findings, and implications. They demonstrated how analyzing qualitative research studies can enhance our ability to critically evaluate findings, understand their strengths and limitations, and determine their applicability to practice decisions.

References

1. Bernhardsson S, Samsson KS, Johansson K, Öberg B, Larsson MEH. A preference for dialogue: Exploring the influence of patient preferences on clinical decision making and treatment in primary care physiotherapy. *Eur J Physiother.* 2019;21(2):107–114. doi:10.1080/21679169.2018.1496474.
2. Joyce C, Keysor J, Stevans J, Ready K, Roseen EJ, Saper RB. Beyond the pain: A qualitative study exploring the physical therapy experience in patients with chronic low back pain. *Physiother Theory Pract.* 2023;39(4):803–813. doi:10.1080/09593985.2022.2029650.
3. Cavazos-Rehg PA, Zewdie K, Krauss MJ, Sowles SJ. "No high like a brownie high": A content analysis of edible marijuana tweets. *Am J Health Promot.* 2018;32(4):880–886. Available from: https://search.ebscohost.com/login.aspx?direct=true&db=s3h&AN=129172845&site=ehost-live
4. Saper RB, Lemaster C, Delitto A, Sherman KJ, Herman PM, Sadikova E et al. Yoga, physical therapy, or education for chronic low back pain: A randomized noninferiority trial. *Ann Intern Med.* 2017;167(2):85–94. doi:10.7326/M16-2579.
5. Polit DF, Beck CT. Generalization in quantitative and qualitative research: Myths and strategies. *Int J Nurs Stud.* 2010;47(11):1451–1458. doi:10.1016/j.ijnurstu.2010.06.004.

PART 3

Understanding Review Studies and Practice Guidelines

Part 3 discusses review studies and their pivotal role in evidence-based practice. Recall that review studies are a special sort of research study – a study of studies where findings from several studies are summarized, analyzed, and synthesized.

Chapter 12 uses traditional narrative reviews as a basic review type that contrasts with systematic reviews. The chapter delineates the crucial distinctions between the two types of reviews, which are central for comprehending the various levels of evidence in health research. The chapter discusses the strengths and potential biases associated with each type of review and provides readers with the tools needed to critically assess their quality. The chapter closes by describing the different levels of evidence professionals use to gauge the quality of evidence offered with different study designs and identifies the systematic review as a "gold standard" with respect to the methodological transparency and rigor needed to limit biases and enhance quality.

Chapter 13 focuses on the critical analysis of systematic reviews. It introduces a structured approach to reading these reviews analytically through a set of 10 questions used to critically analyze the methods of data collection, criteria for study selection, analysis, and the implications of the findings. This chapter is useful for researchers, clinicians, and policymakers who rely on systematic reviews to inform their decisions by helping them assess the quality and applicability of the evidence.

Chapter 14 transitions from the evaluation of evidence to its application in the form of practice guidelines. It explores how systematic reviews may be used to inform practice guidelines that inform clinical decision-making and policy. This chapter discusses the development of guidelines, the importance of regular updates to reflect new evidence, and how these guidelines can be tailored to meet diverse clinical situations and client needs.

DOI: 10.4324/9781003595663-14

12

UNDERSTANDING NARRATIVE AND SYSTEMATIC REVIEWS

Overview of review studies

Our collective knowledge of health issues advances step by step with each new primary study. However, findings from these studies often remain scattered across diverse research publications and research teams. Moreover, the nature and quality of these findings will vary depending on the methods used to collect and analyze data.

As more and more studies are presented in our increasingly crowded information environment, the task of sorting through, critically appraising, comparing, and interpreting their findings is challenging for the busy practitioner. Instead, health professionals will turn to review studies that compare, combine, and report on a set of primary studies.

The next Chapter discusses the critical analysis of *systematic* reviews and *meta-analysis* of primary studies. Systematic reviews limit bias and sit at the apex of the *hierarchy of evidence*. These high-quality review studies are valuable for informing evidence-based guidelines (see Chapter 14) and practice decisions.

Types of review studies – narrative and systematic

As primary studies proliferate, so does the number and variety of review studies. Review studies divide into numerous types and subtypes, with each type taking a somewhat different approach to fulfill their specific aims. For instance, one examination of the review studies available identified 14 different types [1], while another described seven broad review families with over 40 sub-families (Box 12.1).

For current purposes we limit the discussion to the two most contrasting review types – the traditional narrative review and the systematic review. Narrative reviews offer a descriptive summary of research in some areas of health and illness, providing what is essentially an expert's view on a particular health topic. Systematic reviews mainly seek to inform practice decisions, often by pooling and analyzing findings from other studies. Systematic reviews (and its subtypes) serve as a gold standard for review studies designed to shape professional practice.

DOI: 10.4324/9781003595663-15

BOX 12.1 REVIEW FAMILIES

One classification identified seven review families – traditional, systematic, reviews of reviews, rapid reviews, qualitative reviews, mixed methods reviews, and purpose-specific reviews. [2] These families encompass a range of purposes and methodologies. As discussed below, systematic reviews serve to inform practice decisions and offer a model of transparency in characterizing the methods used to select, appraise, and analyze studies under review.

Narrative reviews deviate from systematic reviews in another central way – they mostly bypass any description of the methods used to conduct the review. The Results section immediately follows the Introduction. There is no explicit description of how the studies being reviewed were selected and appraised for quality, or how findings from these studies are collected and analyzed. This leaves narrative reviews open to various biases. For instance, the review might overlook important articles or emphasize results that affirm the author's pre-existing ideas – e.g., selection bias and confirmation bias (see Appendix B).

This lack of transparency makes assessing the quality of the review difficult. They may be judged by the status and influence of its authors, its clarity and coherence, or whether its conclusions correspond with your own. A narrative review offers what is, in effect, an "expert opinion" about what the evidence suggests about the subject of the review.

In contrast, systematic reviews are explicit in the methods used to arrive at a summary and synthesis of their results. Systematic reviews describe the criteria used to select studies for review. Systematic reviews include the protocol used to critically appraise these studies and report the results of the appraisal. When combined with a meta-analysis, systematic reviews will include a protocol for pooling results to construct a "meta"- statistic or "meta"-synthesis.

Systematic reviews are widely seen as the standard for transparency and limiting bias in reviews. Their transparency allows them to be audited for quality and replicated by others, enhancing the reliability, credibility, and applicability of their results. Systematic reviews serve as the "gold standard" for studies that aim to inform evidence-based practice.

Strengths and limitations of review studies

Review studies analyze findings from numerous primary studies, many of which use different modes of data collection and analysis. Review studies are less subject to random variation or unusual findings from any single primary study. Consequently, review studies tend to be more reliable, can represent different populations, and carry more weight than individual studies.

Review studies also vary in terms of their specific aims. Narrative reviews will provide an overview of research on a topic without describing how studies were selected, appraised, or analyzed. In this respect, they offer an "expert opinion" about a particular health topic. This review might still offer the most informed view on a topic, especially where evidence from rigorous primary studies is unavailable.

In contrast, systematic reviews aim to consolidate evidence to help inform practice decisions. Systematic reviews are more reliable, specific, and generalizable than other review types, and serve as a model for analyzing and communicating evidence for practitioners.

Recap

This chapter discussed how review studies help us make sense of the evidence produced by several primary studies on a specific topic in health research. It described how traditional, *narrative* reviews present a summary of evidence from various studies without, however, identifying how these studies were selected, appraised, compared, and analyzed. This lack of transparency leaves narrative reviews open to numerous research biases. Traditional narrative reviews offer what is, in effect, an expert's opinion on the topic.

The chapter contrasts narrative reviews with *systematic* reviews. Whereas narrative reviews lack transparency, systematic reviews are explicit in describing the methods they use to conduct the review. These methods involve a description of how studies were selected and appraised and how the findings were analyzed, and the results presented. This transparency is designed to limit biases in the systematic review. In this regard, systematic reviews serve as the "gold standard" for research evidence. The chapter concludes by identifying the strengths and limitations of these two contrasting types of review studies.

References

1. Grant MJ, Booth A. A typology of reviews: An analysis of 14 review types and associated methodologies. *Health Info Libr J*. 2009;26(2):91–108. doi:10.1111/j.1471-1842.2009.00848.x.
2. Sutton A, Clowes M, Preston L, Booth A. Meeting the review family: Exploring review types and associated information retrieval requirements. *Health Info Libr J*. 2019;36(3):202–222. doi:10.1111/hir.12276.

13

ANALYZING SYSTEMATIC REVIEWS

Analytical questions for systematic reviews

The question of an article's relevance (Q1) and research design (Q2) are basic to all peer-reviewed studies, including systematic reviews. Q1 and Q2 may be answered during inspectional reading.

Q1. Is the review study relevant?
Q2. What type(s) of studies were systematically reviewed?

Once the first two questions are answered, three questions of the methods and three questions of the results that are specific to review studies will assist in critically analyzing the results. The three questions to ask in the Methods section are:

Q3. What inclusion and exclusion criteria were used to select studies for review?
Q4. How were the selected studies assessed for quality?
Q5. How were data extracted and analyzed?

The Results section describes the findings derived from the methods. Further questions arise regarding how to characterize the results

Q6. How were selected studies characterized?
Q7. How was the quality and heterogeneity of the selected studies characterized?
Q8. What major findings were emphasized in the narrative summary or meta-analysis?

Answers serve to deepen one's understanding of the results, their strengths, limitations, and implications for EBP. This returns us to the final two questions that are asked of the Discussion section that concludes all peer-reviewed articles:

DOI: 10.4324/9781003595663-16

Q9. What were the strengths and limitations of the review?

Q10. What were the implications of the review for research and practice?

We elaborate on the ten questions used to analyze systematic reviews.

Inspectional reading

Q1   Is the review study relevant?

As with all peer-reviewed articles, readers will address the question of relevance during the inspectional phase of reading. Inspecting the title and abstract will enable the reader to identify the key health outcomes, exposures, or experiences being explored, along with study objectives. Their alignment with the reader's aim will influence the assessment of the study's relevance.

Q2   What type(s) of studies were systematically reviewed?

Not all systematic reviews are same, and the type of review also factors into the question of relevance. With practice, you will develop skills in distinguishing between different types of reviews. First, the title usually identifies a review as systematic

- Social determinants of multimorbidity patterns: A *systematic* review [1]
- The association between food insecurity and dietary outcomes in university students: A *systematic* review [2].

Based on their titles, these systematic reviews are not restricting the review to studies that use a certain research design. Often, however, systematic reviews limit the review to primary studies that use a specific research design. Again, this is often clear from the title

- Barriers and facilitators associated with the adoption of and adherence to a Mediterranean style diet in adults: A systematic review of *published observational and qualitative studies* [3].
- Lifestyle interventions to improve glycemic control in adults with type 2 diabetes living in low-and-middle income countries: A systematic review and *meta-analysis of randomized controlled trials* (RCTs) [4].

The first review study targets observational and qualitative studies; the second limits the review to RCTs. Narrowing the focus to studies that use the same design enhances the comparability and interpretation of the results. Some "umbrella" reviews systematically review multiple other systematic reviews (Box 13.1).

The types of study designs included in the review will indicate the type of evidence the review will produce, and potentially its overall value to the reader. Reviews of RCTs attempt to consolidate evidence on the effects of interventions on health outcomes. Reviews of observational studies will identify patterns of relationships among exposures

---

BOX 13.1 REVIEW OF REVIEWS

Although review studies primarily analyze and synthesize results from primary research, reviews are increasingly able to analyze and synthesize results of other systematic reviews – "systematic reviews of systematic reviews". These are sometimes called "umbrella" reviews. Umbrella reviews may also include a meta-analysis to synthesize findings of numerous systematic reviews.

---

and outcomes to suggest how specific exposures may reduce or increase the risk of certain health outcomes occurring. Reviews of qualitative studies will illuminate the perspectives and experiences of certain groups as expressed in terms of larger themes. Broader reviews that include various study designs often aim to describe the current landscape of research in a specific area, and to identify promising areas for future research.

Systematic reviews may also include a "meta-" analysis or a "meta-" synthesis, where statistics or themes are analyzed and captured in a set of "meta" statistics or "meta" themes:

- Weight loss in short-term interventions for physical activity and nutrition among adults with overweight or obesity: A systematic review and meta-analysis [5].
- Patient and carer experience of living with a pressure injury: A meta-synthesis of qualitative studies [6].

Meta-analyses and meta-syntheses provide an additional component to systematic reviews, strengthening the reliability and comprehensiveness of the base of evidence used to inform health practice. Both are discussed below.

Reading the methods

Q3   What inclusion and exclusion criteria were used to select studies for review?

Review studies use online search tools to locate and identify articles to review. Systematic reviews, however, differ in their explicit description of how searches are conducted and what articles will be included and excluded in the review. They will identify the keywords used and databases searched, the criteria for excluding and including articles, and the process of screening irrelevant articles and keeping relevant ones for review.

For example, a systematic review of studies about food insecurity and dietary outcomes described databases searched and search terms as follows

> The full search was conducted in 9 electronic databases in July 2020, including MEDLINE, EMBASE, ERIC, PsycINFO, GlobalHealth, CINAHL, CENTRAL, Scopus, and Web of Science. The search terms for MEDLINE are shown in Table 1.... [2]

The study was focused on dietary outcomes among university students who were food insecure, and data about this might appear in separate governmental reports rather than in peer-reviewed articles. To find relevant studies from the gray literature and to limit publication bias (Appendix B), the study also used "Google Scholar" and "Mednar".

A comprehensive online search across several databases will return myriad titles, most of which may not be relevant for the review. Criteria for including or excluding titles are defined and used to screen titles. For instance, a systematic review of RCTs on the effects of creatine on performance identified specific attributes of RCTs that were to be met for studies to be included in the review:

a description of strength performance at baseline and following supplementation or placebo with a double-blind randomization, and the duration of exercise when performance was measured had to be less than 3 min.

The more well-defined the eligibility criteria, the more comparable the results of the different studies will be, facilitating a more credible synthesis of their findings.

No matter how well defined at the outset, searches of multiple databases will flag many more articles than are actually relevant for the review. Thus, a systematic review will also define the process of sorting through and inspecting hundreds of titles, abstract, and the full text of articles to identify only those that meet the eligibility criteria is also defined.

For instance, a search for studies on the effects of creatine supplementation on performance initially identified 1,265 titles and abstracts, most of which were irrelevant to the primary aim. Two researchers independently screened titles and abstracts for inclusion, while a third researcher was available to help resolve differences in screening decisions as they arise. This resembles the "analyst triangulation" used in qualitative studies.

The process of selecting articles is analogous to the process of selecting the sample in primary studies. Explicitly defining the various components of the selection process enables others to assess how comprehensive, inclusive and trustworthy the selection process was. Once selected, studies under review are each critically appraised for quality.

Q4   How were the selected studies assessed for quality?

Systematic reviews use critical appraisal tools to assess selected primary studies for quality and risk of bias. These tools often appear as checklists that contain several items used to grade each study (Box 13.2). For instance, the checklist may include items regarding the sampling strategy, reliability and validity of measurements, confounding variables, participant attrition, and other sources of bias. Each item may be graded as "Yes", "No", "Unclear", or "Not applicable". Scores on each item are tallied to provide an overall assessment of quality of each study reviewed – e.g., "low", "medium" or "high".

It is worthwhile noting how studies being reviewed score in terms of quality assessment. As a reader you would have greater confidence in evidence from reviews of high-quality studies, than from reviews of low or modest quality studies. In fact, whether it is more fruitful to focus on a few high-quality studies rather than many more studies of modest or low quality remains an open question.

The Results section often presents a table that shows the results of the appraisal of each study. From the table you can consider the quality of studies under review and what it means for understanding and the overall results.

BOX 13.2 APPRAISAL TOOLS AND CHECKLISTS

There are various appraisal tools available to gauge the quality and risk of bias for studies that use different research designs – e.g., cross-sectional, cohort, RCTs, and qualitative. Several national and international teams of experts collaborate to develop and maintain these checklists – e.g., the Cochrane Library, the Joanna Briggs Institute (JBI), and the CONSORT group. Checklists offer a standard tool for researchers to assess the quality of studies under review in terms of methods of data collection and analysis.

Q5   How were data extracted and analyzed?

Extracting data. Systematic reviews will define and describe how and what findings were extracted from each article – e.g., author, year, research design, study population, outcome measures, and other attributes of the primary studies pertinent to the specific review. For instance, a systematic review of studies of the relationship between food insecurity and diet among university students reports that the following data were extracted from the studies under review:

> … author, year of publication, country of the study, research aims, study design, measures of exposures and outcomes, data analysis, demographics of participants, description of the setting, food security status, dietary outcomes, the association between food insecurity and dietary outcomes, and implications of the study [2].

To enhance its reliability and limit bias, the extraction process is often undertaken by two members of the research team: "data extraction was carried out using a standardized extraction form and conducted independently by 2 researchers, with disagreements resolved by a third researcher" [7].

A similar process is involved for extracting non-numeric data from qualitative studies, though it typically requires additional judgment and interpretation on the part of the researchers. Like the structured coding process used in qualitative studies, inconsistencies in the extraction of data from each study can be limited by the use of pre-defined data-extraction forms.

Data Analysis. To prepare data for analysis, systematic reviews extract and organize data drawn from each study under review. Based on this, systematic reviews will provide a narrative summary of the studies being reviewed (Box 13.3). This summary will characterize studies being reviewed by their key attributes – e.g., study designs, population, measures, and key outcomes.

- For data analysis, a narrative synthesis and summary of the different methods of identifying patterns and their association with different social determinants were described… [1]
- The statistical significance of the differences in dietary outcomes between food-secure and -insecure students was also summarized [2].

BOX 13.3   NARRATIVE SUMMARIES

A narrative summary provides a comprehensive description of the methods and findings of studies being reviewed. It may also involve a qualitative synthesis of the results, describing how they vary in terms of study designs, populations, and outcomes. This enables them to characterize the current state of our knowledge of a topic, and where further research is needed to expand our knowledge and understanding.

Systematic reviews are often only able to supply a narrative summary of the research in an area, often because research on the topic is limited and the methods used to study it are so varied that identifying common statistical trends or themes is impossible. For other areas where several studies use similar research protocols, it becomes feasible to pool the data from these studies to generate an encompassing "meta" statistic. Thus, the systematic review may include a "meta-analysis" that combines findings from various studies being reviewed.

Meta-analyses of quantitative findings

If the data extracted from primary studies are well-defined and comparable, systematic reviews may also involve a meta-analysis of research findings. The analysis will extract and pool data from each study – e.g., sample sizes, standard deviations, confidence intervals, and effect size statistics – to generate a set of meta-statistics about the relationships between exposures and key health outcomes. Pooled or aggregated results based on findings from several primary studies is the product of a meta-analysis (Box 13.4).

Typically, the article will describe the parameters surrounding how major outcomes will be meta-analyzed – how findings from different studies will be standardized and brought together to compute a pooled result. For instance, the meta-analysis of the effects of creatine on upper limb performance would combine results from several studies that compare relative change in limb performance for intervention and control groups:

… we conducted a third group of meta-analyses with the relative percent changes (T1-T0)/T0 for both groups… – the creatine supplementation and control groups [8].

Another study extracted findings from primary studies on the effects of physical activity on risk of infection, severity, and mortality from COVID-19 – "RR [relative risk] values were pooled when comparing the inactive (reference group) versus active categories in relation to COVID-19 outcomes" [9].

Another key product of a meta-analysis is an assessment of how consistent or inconsistent were the findings from the different studies being reviewed.

Consistent and inconsistent results – heterogeneity. As you would expect, results will not be identical across different studies. These different results are a product of numerous differences among studies that use the same basic design. Sample populations vary, measures used might be different, or the interventions differ as they are adapted to specific research settings. Study findings will vary correspondingly. A meta-analysis will assess the extent of inconsistency or *heterogeneity* among study findings from studies being reviewed. An analysis of this heterogeneity is included in the meta-analysis – the I^2 statistic is commonly used to quantify this heterogeneity.

> We assessed statistical heterogeneity (i.e., variability resulting from differences in the study effects) in pooled estimates by examining I statistics and p-values. We considered I values of 0% to 40% to indicate unimportant heterogeneity, 30% to 60% to indicate moderate heterogeneity, 50% to 90% to indicate substantial heterogeneity, and 75% to 100% to indicate considerable heterogeneity [5].

Considerable heterogeneity suggests that the findings from different studies vary significantly and may be highly sensitive to small differences in the methods of these different studies. This lowers the reliability of the pooled result of the meta-analysis.

BOX 13.4 STANDALONE META-ANALYSES

Whenever you see a title that reads as a "systematic review and meta-analysis of..." you will know that a meta-analysis is included with the systematic review. However, you may encounter a meta-analysis that is not attached to a systematic review. A standalone meta-analysis will skip the search for titles and description of the topical literature, and, instead, collect and analyze data from two or more datasets.

Meta-syntheses of qualitative themes

Just as numeric data may be extracted from quantitative studies for analysis, non-numeric text data may be extracted from qualitative studies, pooled, and analyzed in developing a meta-synthesis of themes. For instance, a meta-synthesis of findings from qualitative studies of families with chronically ill children involved line-by-line coding of the results and organizing and analyzing these codes to construct descriptive and analytical themes:

> first the free line-by-line coding of findings in primary studies and creation of "free codes"; second the organization of these "free codes" into related areas to construct descriptive themes; and third, the development of analytical themes [10].

The synthesis involves describing and employing methods similar to those used in primary qualitative studies – e.g., line-by-line coding, organizing codes, categorizing codes into themes and subthemes. In the case of meta-syntheses, data are drawn from various qualitative studies to distill broader themes.

Reading the results

Questions about methods (Q3, Q4, and Q5) ask about the process of data collection and analysis. Questions about results (Q6, Q7, and Q8) seek to understand the results of the data collection and analysis process.

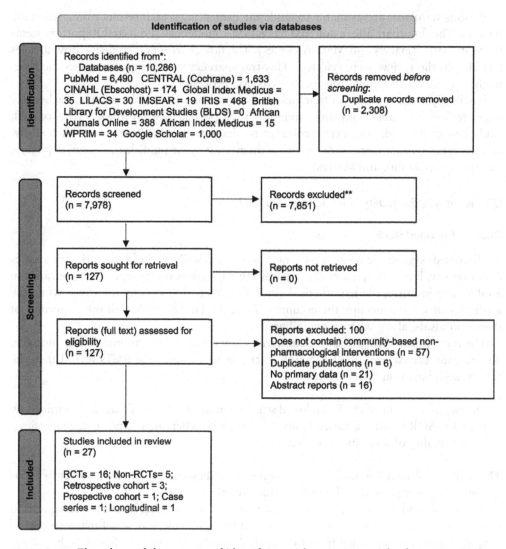

FIGURE 13.1   Flowchart of the process of identifying and screening articles for review [11].

Q6   How were selected studies characterized?

The process of selecting studies in a systematic review is usually captured in a flowchart such as the one shown in Figure 13.1 [11].

In this example, the systematic review searched 12 databases and reference lists to identify primary studies on non-pharmacological, community-based interventions for pregnant women with gestational diabetes. The search identified 7,978 non-duplicate records, of which 7,851 were excluded based on their titles and abstracts. The full text of the 127 remaining articles were read, 100 of which were excluded for various reasons. This left 27 studies included in the final synthesis. Of the 27 selected studies, 16 were RCTs, 5 were non-RCTS, and 6 were observational designs. The nature of the evidence supplied by these designs will differ, as will the conclusions drawn from them [11].

Various standards are available to guide the presenting search results from systematic reviews. The flowchart above adhered to PRISMA guidelines (Preferred Reporting Items for Systematic Reviews and Meta-Analyses). The flowchart serves to define how articles included in the review were selected. This transparency enables one to assess the thoroughness, biases, and limitations of the selection process.

Finally, systematic reviews often include a sprawling table to characterize each study under review. The table, sometimes spanning multiple pages, will include a row for each study being reviewed, and several columns to characterize key attributes of each study, and the types of data were extracted from them – e.g., year published, design, exposure, outcome, population, and key results.

Q7   What was the quality of the selected studies?

Quality of selected studies

As discussed, systematic reviews use checklists to critically appraise the primary studies under review. For instance, a systematic review will report the results of the appraisal in a table. For instance, the hypothetical studies under review occupy the rows, while the attributes of interest occupy the columns (Table 13.1). The table will offer specifics of these appraisals, along with an overall grade.

The text surrounding the table summarizes key results of the appraisal. For instance, a systematic review used the CONSORT criteria to appraise the RCTs included in the review, and, based on the criteria,

> Quality assessment of the 53 included studies reporting T0 and T1 data, as outlined by the CONSORT criteria, varied from 22% to 65%, where higher percentage implies a higher quality of scientific reporting" [8].

The review also characterized the percentage of studies that reported a conflict of interest, funding sources, or that did not provide the information.

Readers should note the nature and quality of the studies being reviewed. The question lingers about whether readers are better served by systematic reviews of many studies of low, moderate, and high quality or by a critical analysis of fewer studies of high quality.

TABLE 13.1 Results of the reviewer's appraisal of RCTs – risk of bias checklist

Citation	Random assign	Blinding	Attrition	...	Other biases	Overall grade
Kumar et al (2024)	No	Yes, double	No	No	No	Low risk
Sanchez et al (2017)	Yes	No	Unclear	No	Yes	Med. risk
...	Unclear	Unclear	Unclear	Yes	Yes	High risk
Ammar et al. (2019)	No	Yes	Yes	No	Yes	Med risk
Dunmore et al (2011)	Unclear	No	Unclear	Yes	Yes	High risk

The citations are hypothetical.

*Q8   What major findings were emphasized in the narrative summary or
meta-analysis?*

Once the quality and basic attributes of the studies under review have been characterized,
review studies will report the key findings presented in these studies. Systematic reviews
provide a narrative summary of the results of these studies. As discussed, some reviews
also include a meta-analysis of findings. Most basically, they offer a summary of the results in narrative form.

The narrative summary

A narrative summary offers a basic description of the studies under review – e.g., their
research design, quality, and major findings. For instance, a systematic review of observational studies on the effects of student food insecurity summarizes findings on dietary
intake

> Significantly lower intakes of total fruits and vegetables among food-insecure students
> was observed in 5 out of 6 studies. [30, 33, 39, 41, 44] ... Significantly higher intake of
> sweets or added sugars among food-insecure students was observed in 1 out of 7 stud-
> ies [38]. Significantly higher intake of added sugars from sugar-sweetened beverages
> was observed in 1 out of 3 studies [38]. No significant differences were reported in the
> consumption of fat ($n = 2$) [32, 42] discretionary choices such as snack chips and instant
> noodles ($n = 2$) [32, 42] alcohol ($n = 3$) [30, 32, 36] and fiber ($n = 3$). [30, 38, 44] [2].

The passage indicates which associations were supported by the evidence and which ones
were not. Several studies showed support for an association between food insecurity and
fruit and vegetable intake. There is less evidence to support a relationship between food
insecurity and the consumption of added sugar and fat.

The narrative summary provides the health professional with a straightforward picture of the current state of the evidence on a health topic or question. The summary will
highlight key findings, the quality of the studies reviewed, and the limitations or gaps in
what we know. The narrative summary is often a precursor to a "meta-analysis" which
will aggregate and synthesize results to generate a set of "meta"- statistics from quantitative studies under review [12].

Analyzing findings from a meta-analysis

As discussed, systematic reviews may also include a meta-analysis of quantitative data extracted from the studies being reviewed. Tables and figures are commonly used to present
findings from several studies being reviewed, along with a pooled statistic used to estimate the overall association between an exposure or intervention on the health outcome.
These tables are often accompanied by a forest plot. For instance, Table 13.2 are commonly found in meta-analysis, and are often accompanied by a forest plot (Box 13.5).

Table 13.2 shows the results of a meta-analysis of six studies that examined the effects of running on lower limb cartilage [12]. Column 1 provides citations of the primary
studies being reviewed. Columns 2 and 3 provide the mean and standard deviations for
media tibial cartilage volume at pre-run and post-run. Each study is assigned a weight
(column 4), based on the sample size and standard deviation of each. Column 5 presents

TABLE 13.2 Pooled results of studies examining T2 relaxation values pre- and post-running

1 Study	2 Pre-run mean (SD)	3 Post-run mean (SD)	4 Weight	5 SMD, 95% CI
Esculier [13]	34.80 (7.05)	34.60 (7.91)	15.5%	−0.03 (−0.90; 0.85)
Esculier [13]	34.10 (4.61)	31.50 (5.17)	15.0%	−0.51 (−1.40; 0.39)
Gatti [14]	36.61 (2.85)	34.35 (3.16)	18.6%	−0.73 (−1.50; 0.04)
Subburaj [15]	23.92 (1.75)	21.12 (1.66)	20.3%	−1.61 (−2.33; −0.89)*
Cha [16]	30.85 (6.05)	28.43 (4.28)	15.1%	−0.44 (−1.33; 0.45)
Cha [16]	23.17 (6.63)	23.02 (6.65)	15.5%	−0.02 (−0.90; 0.85)
Total				−0.59 (−1.10; −0.08)*

Heterogeneity: I^2 = 55% (0%; 82%); * p ≤ 0.05.
Adapted from "Fig 3 Forest plot of data for pooling T2 relaxation values immediately following running."
Data from [12].

the standardized mean difference (SMD) to indicate the size of the effect of running on cartilage volume (Appendix F).

The minus sign indicates that volume was reduced pre-run to post-run. The accompanying number is a point estimate to indicate the extent of the reduction in standard deviations (95% CIs are provided next to the estimate). While only one of the primary studies was statistically significant on its own, the combined findings from these studies show a significant reduction in cartilage volume, with an effect size of −0.59 standard deviations (the 95% CI ranging from −1.10 to −0.08). An effect size of −0.59 standard deviations is considered moderate.

Finally, a heterogeneity statistic is shown in the table – i.e., Heterogeneity: I^2 = 55% (0%; 82%); * p ≤ 0.05. The statistic estimates the likelihood that variation in study findings is due to real differences rather than random chance (Box 13.5). While some variation due to chance is expected, the heterogeneity statistic helps us discern how much of this variation is due to real (not random) differences in study characteristics (sample sizes, populations, methods, quality). An I^2 = 55% is considered as "moderate" to "substantial" degree of heterogeneity or inconsistency among studies.

BOX 13.5 CONSISTENCY AND HETEROGENEITY OF FINDINGS

Systematic reviews and meta-analyses assess the degree of consistency or variation (heterogeneity) in the findings of studies being reviewed. Meta-analyses often use forest plots to show this variation.

In plots A and B the total point-estimates are the same – both favor control over treatment. In plot A, however, there is considerable overlap in the confidence intervals of the studies and the point estimates more or less align. This suggests a degree of consistency in the results. In contrast, the results shown in Plot B are more scattered, and some findings favor the intervention, some favor the control. Readers will be more confident when results from the various studies being reviewed are consistent rather than heterogeneous.

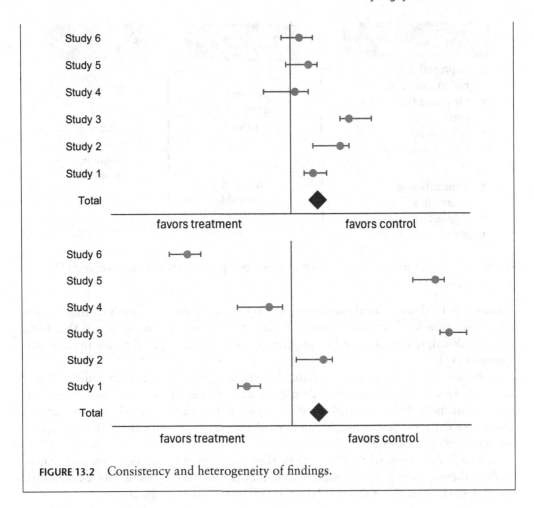

FIGURE 13.2   Consistency and heterogeneity of findings.

Analyzing findings from a qualitative meta-synthesis

Much like a meta-analysis of quantitative studies, a meta-synthesis of qualitative studies combines non-numeric data from each primary study to produce a meta-synthesis of these themes. Once data are extracted from each study, the process of synthesizing results of qualitative studies parallels the process of aggregating results of quantitative studies in a meta-analysis.

For instance, the passage below illustrates an approach to synthesizing text from qualitative studies exploring participants' perspectives of short message service (SMS) designed to promote physical activity

> Two researchers (JG, KH) independently completed line-by-line coding of relevant data and developed initial codes to summarize ideas presented in the text. These were then compared, and new collated codes were created to capture the agreed meaning of the portions of text, referring each time to their meaning in the context of the original study (see Box 13.6). Final codes were grouped into descriptive themes to summarise the original findings of the data [17].

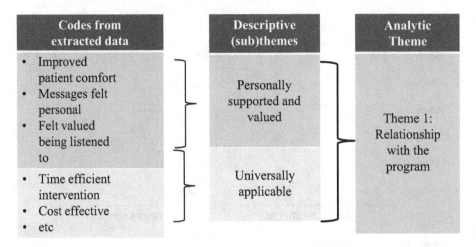

FIGURE 13.3   Transforming codes to themes – user perspectives on SMS interventions [17].

From these 10 descriptive themes, the meta-synthesis identified 5 analytic themes that cut across various descriptive themes. Figure 13.3 illustrates the sequence that links codes to descriptive themes and descriptive themes to an analytical theme in the meta-synthesis [17].

Codes are one step removed from the data itself, capturing specific qualities and perspectives. Descriptive themes provide a descriptive summary of the main content and meaning of the coded data. Analytic themes look below surface descriptions to capture underlying patterns, deeper insight, and broader perspectives on findings that cut across multiple descriptive themes.

The table shows one of the five analytic themes captured in the meta-synthesis. These analytic themes from a meta-synthesis should be scrutinized as one would a qualitative research study – assessing the credibility and trustworthiness of the themes.

BOX 13.6   IS A SYNTHESIS OF QUALITATIVE STUDIES EVEN POSSIBLE?

Qualitative studies aim to gain a holistic understanding of people's experiences, and this often entails anchoring results in their specific, material, and social context. Qualitative studies aim to capture the particulars that characterize experiences and perspectives. Some might argue that the process of extracting and synthesizing qualitative data itself defeats the basic purpose of providing a grounded, holistic perspective – text data when removed from their context loses some of its complexity and can take on different meanings. On the other hand, uncovering themes that cut across diverse groups and settings strengthens our sense that the experiences these themes capture are authentic and common.

Reading the discussion

Q9   What were the strengths and limitations of the review?

Systematic reviews compile evidence from numerous studies, making them less prone to the effects of random variation present in individual studies. By aggregating findings from multiple studies, review studies limit the effects of skewed or extreme data so the results are more reliable than of those of single primary studies. Further, by drawing on more diverse study populations, results of systematic reviews are more broadly applicable.

Systematic reviews also include a critical appraisal of the primary studies included in the review, enabling one to gauge the quality of these studies. In addition to critically appraising the quality of primary studies, systematic reviews identify how consistent studies are with respect to their methods and results. The more consistent the results, the more confident we are that a relationship is real. Health professionals will consider both the quality and consistency of the studies being reviewed when assessing the implications of the evidence for research and practice.

Q10   What were the implications of the review for research and practice?

Health professionals should meet the results of reviews with the same skepticism that they maintain when analyzing primary studies. First, systematic reviews often include studies that use various research designs or are of poor quality or produce results that are highly inconsistent. Poor quality and inconsistent results may be valuable for identifying research gaps, but they are of lesser importance for informing practice decisions.

Finally, the results of systematic reviews typically carry greater weight than those of single studies (Figure 13.3), largely for reasons identified above – they are more reliable and less vulnerable to biases or skewed findings that can appear in individual primary studies. Hence, they tend to have a larger impact on evidence-based decisions. Moreover, high quality systematic reviews play a critical role in shaping and updating practice guidelines that are foundational for evidence-based practice see Chapter 14).

Research design, risk of bias, and levels of evidence

Research designs are commonly ranked according to their risk of bias and their potential to yield valid and reliable evidence. This pyramid of evidence is depicted in Figure 13.4.

Expert opinion sits at the base of the pyramid. It is surely more valid than a less-informed, non-expert opinion based on idiosyncratic, cherry-picked evidence that confirms a pre-existing view. Expert opinion is superior to the constant noise of misinformation and partial information that increasingly drowns out the signal. Expert opinion is useful in areas where more clarifying research evidence is unavailable. Expert opinions on a health issue are garnered from personal consultations, commentaries, case-studies, or traditional narrative reviews (see Box 13.7). Nonetheless, the risk of bias remains significant, and the validity of expert opinion is hard to gauge without transparency surrounding the evidence supporting them.

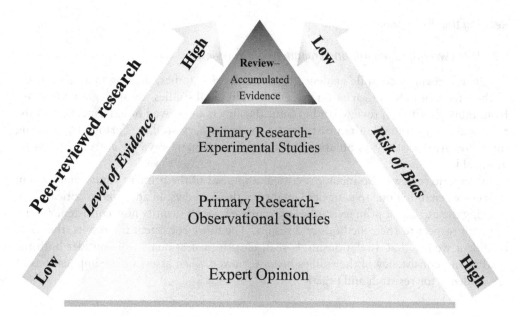

FIGURE 13.4 Research designs, risk of bias, and levels of evidence.

BOX 13.7 IN DEFENSE OF EXPERT OPINION

Although "expert opinion" sits at the base of the pyramid, readers should also consider that the opinions of experts are likely to be much more informed, reliable, carefully considered, and trustworthy than the opinion of the lesser trained and experienced non-expert. In fact, health professionals routinely consult with other experts for a second opinion. Further, the traditional peer-reviewed article expresses the views of experts on the research team and has been vetted by outside peers.

Expert opinion falls just below observational studies on the evidence pyramid. Although the figure does not include them, qualitative studies are sometimes situated just above expert opinion and below observational designs (Box 13.8). Observational designs sit between expert opinion and clinical trials and RCTs – controlled studies where the risk of biases is minimized. Observational studies provide evidence that supports an association (e.g., positive or negative, strong or weak) between exposures and outcomes. They help to characterize associations between exposures that are detrimental or beneficial to health and wellness. Nonetheless, observational studies observe phenomena in their natural environment and hence do not control the complex array of covariates that might confound the results. High-quality observational studies can limit, but not eliminate, the effects of these confounders.

Experimental studies – e.g., clinical trials and RCTs – serve as the gold standard for primary studies with regard to limiting biases in assessing the effects of an intervention on health outcomes. With experimental studies variables are controlled, and the effects of the intervention on health outcomes can be more clearly specified. In turn, this can help us manage and control these outcomes. While this gives the experiment strong "internal validity", it may compromise "external validity" where generalizing from controlled experimental settings to complex real-world settings, or from small, homogeneous populations to other diverse populations often becomes challenging.

Systematic reviews and meta-analyses of RCTs sit at the apex of the pyramid. Systematic reviews enable results from multiple RCTs to be compared and synthesized. As we have seen, results from different studies may be inconsistent and the populations, study designs, and findings will vary. Systematic reviews and meta-analyses compile and harmonize findings from several studies, rather than a single study that might deviate from the others. As always, however, it is advisable to remain skeptical even of systematic reviews where the quality and consistency of primary studies being reviewed may be poor or highly variable.

BOX 13.8 QUALITATIVE STUDIES AND LEVELS OF EVIDENCE

Conspicuous is the absence of qualitative studies from the hierarchy. Their absence reflects how different qualitative studies are in terms of their research aims and methods, and the findings they produce. They are qualitatively different. The aim is not to specify the effects of a treatment intervention on outcomes. Rather, qualitative studies provide a rich description and deeper understanding of human experiences and perspectives as expressed in particular settings. Results from qualitative designs complement, rather than compete with, results from quantitative designs. Some depictions of the pyramid may include qualitative designs at or near the pyramid's base, providing evidence that is closest to expert opinion. We prefer to leave it out entirely, to suggest the fundamentally different purposes quantitative and qualitative research aims to serve.

Recap

This chapter identified ten questions used to analyze systematic reviews. The answers to these questions illustrate the transparency of systematic reviews with respect to the systematic undertaking of the review itself – selecting and appraising studies for review, extracting and analyzing findings from these studies, and presenting the results.

The chapter also described how systematic reviews help us gauge the quality and consistency of the current evidence on the topic. Consistent results seen across various studies give us greater confidence in the evidence supporting an association. Where appropriate, systematic reviews will pool findings from selected studies in a "meta"-analysis or meta-synthesis of the evidence. These combined results provide an overall estimate of the strength of a relationship or enable us to capture prevailing qualitative themes.

Finally, this chapter discussed the levels of evidence that characterize different research designs. This pyramid of evidence is based on the risk of bias associated with the various research designs. Systematic reviews of RCTs sit at the apex of this pyramid, offering the most current and comprehensive statement of the state of knowledge on a particular topic. These studies serve to inform evidence-based practice guidelines provided for health professionals (Chapter 14).

References

1. Álvarez-Gálvez J, Ortega-Martín E, Carretero-Bravo J, Pérez-Muñoz C, Suárez-Lledó V, Ramos-Fiol B. Social determinants of multimorbidity patterns: A systematic review. *Front Public Health*. 2023;11:1081518. doi:10.3389/fpubh.2023.1081518.
2. Shi Y, Davies A, Allman-Farinelli M. The association between food insecurity and dietary outcomes in university students: A systematic review. *J Acad Nutr Diet*. 2021;121(12):2475–2500.e1. doi:10.1016/j.jand.2021.07.015.
3. Tsofliou F, Vlachos D, Hughes C, Appleton KM. Barriers and facilitators associated with the adoption of and adherence to a Mediterranean style diet in adults: A systematic review of published observational and qualitative studies. *Nutrients*. 2022;14(20):4314. doi:10.3390/nu14204314.
4. O'Donoghue G, O'Sullivan C, Corridan I, Daly J, Finn R, Melvin K, et al. Lifestyle interventions to improve glycemic control in adults with type 2 diabetes living in low-and-middle income countries: A systematic review and meta-analysis of randomized controlled trials (RCTs). *Int J Environ Res Public Health*. 2021;18(12):6273. doi:10.3390/ijerph18126273.
5. Rotunda W, Rains C, Jacobs SR, Ng V, Lee R, Rutledge S, et al. Weight loss in short-term interventions for physical activity and nutrition among adults with overweight or obesity: A systematic review and meta-analysis. *Prev Chronic Dis*. 2024;21:E21. doi:10.5888/pcd21.230347.
6. Burston A, Miles SJ, Fulbrook P. Patient and carer experience of living with a pressure injury: A meta-synthesis of qualitative studies. *J Clin Nurs*. 2023;32(13-14):3233–3247. doi:10.1111/jocn.16431.
7. Pearce M, Garcia L, Abbas A, Strain T, Schuch FB, Golubic R, et al. Association between physical activity and risk of depression: A systematic review and meta-analysis. *JAMA Psychiatry*. 2022;79(6):550–559. doi:10.1001/jamapsychiatry.2022.0609.
8. Lanhers C, Pereira B, Naughton G, Trousselard M, Lesage FX, Dutheil F. Creatine supplementation and upper limb strength performance: A systematic review and meta-analysis. *Sports Med*. 2017;47(1):163–173. doi:10.1007/s40279-016-0571-4.
9. Ezzatvar Y, Ramírez-Rodríguez R, Izquierdo M, García-Hermoso A. Physical activity and risk of infection, severity, and mortality of COVID-19: A systematic review and non-linear dose–response meta-analysis of data from 1,853,610 adults. *Br J Sports Med*. 2022;56(20):1–7. doi:10.1136/bjsports-2022-105733.
10. Leite ACAB, Garcia-Vivar C, Neris RR, Alvarenga W, Nascimento LC. The experience of hope in families of children and adolescents living with chronic illness: A thematic synthesis of qualitative studies. *J Adv Nurs*. 2019;75(12):3246–3262. doi:10.1111/jan.14129.
11. Igwesi-Chidobe CN, Okechi PC, Emmanuel GN, Ozumba BC. Community-based non-pharmacological interventions for pregnant women with gestational diabetes mellitus: A systematic review. *BMC Womens Health*. 2022;22:482. doi:10.1186/s12905-022-02038-9.
12. Khan MCM, O'Donovan J, Charlton JM, Roy JS, Hunt MA, Esculier JF. The influence of running on lower limb cartilage: A systematic review and meta-analysis. *Sports Med*. 2022;52:55–74. doi:10.1007/s40279-021-01533-7.
13. Esculier JF, Jarrett M, Krowchuk NM, Rauscher A, Wiggermann V, Taunton JE, et al. Cartilage recovery in runners with and without knee osteoarthritis: a pilot study. *Knee*. 2019;26:1049–1057.
14. Gatti AA, Noseworthy MD, Stratford PW, Brenneman EC, Totterman S, Tamez-Peña J, et al. Acute changes in knee cartilage transverse relaxation time after running and bicycling. *J Biomech*. 2017;53:171–177.
15. Subburaj K, Kumar D, Souza RB, Alizai H, Li X, Link TM, et al. The acute effect of running on knee articular cartilage and meniscus magnetic resonance relaxation times in young healthy adults. *Am J Sports Med*. 2012;40:2134–2141.
16. Cha JG, Lee JC, Kim HJ, Han JK, Lee EH, Kim YD, et al. Comparison of MRI T2 relaxation changes of knee articular cartilage before and after running between young and old amateur athletes. *Korean J Radiol*. 2012;13:594–601.
17. Grobler JS, Stavric V, Saywell NL. Participant perspectives of automated short messaging service interventions to promote physical activity: A systematic review and thematic synthesis. *Digit Health*. 2022;8:20552076221113705. doi:10.1177/20552076221113705.

14

EVIDENCE REVIEW AND PRACTICE

Overview of evidence review and practice guidelines

Practice guidelines provide a framework for health professionals to make decisions and take actions with respect to their clients and patients. Guidelines are developed by regulatory bodies and professional organizations across diverse health professions (Box 14.1). They capture what subject-matter experts on a topic consider to be the best evidence available on a topic at the time the guideline was created. Guidelines are a central component for evidence-based practice.

BOX 14.1 ORGANIZATIONS FOR HEALTH PROFESSIONS

Health professionals are members of professional organizations that represent their interests, and the interests of the clients they serve. These organizations oversee accreditation of programs designed to educate and socialize future health professionals. They also host journals and conferences that member professionals read and attend to communicate experiences and evidence about current practices. Professional organizations offer key resources to support practice that is evidence-based.

Guidelines offer the flexibility needed for health professionals to tailor their application according to the client's specific needs, preferences, and circumstances. The strength and reliability of the evidence supporting different sets of recommendations varies and is reported for professionals to weigh and consider. Thus, when working with guidelines, the evidence-based practitioner will consider the strength and consistency of the evidence underpinning guideline recommendations as they apply them to unique cases.

Guideline development and updates

The particulars of guideline development vary across professional associations and various regulatory bodies, but the steps involved are generally similar. Taking the process

DOI: 10.4324/9781003595663-17

used to update *Dietary Guidelines for Americans* (DGAs) to illustrate, the U.S. Departments of Health and Human Services (HHS) and Agriculture (USDA) undertake a 5-step process to update the DGAs every 5 years and to provide clear information to the public (allowing for public participation in the process).

1 **Step 1 – Identify the Scientific Questions.** After a consultation with experts and the public, scientific questions are identified that shape the examination of recent evidence. Questions are prioritized based on relevance, importance to the public, and health impact.
2 **Step 2 – Appoint the Advisory Committee.** A team of experts is appointed to the advisory committee to review the evidence. There are also subcommittees formed, including members with expertise in different areas. The subcommittees convene to analyze scientific evidence and to provide advice for updating the guidelines.
3 **Step 3 – Advisory Committee Reviews Scientific Evidence.** The committee members collaborate to develop evidence review protocols, to synthesize evidence and present the scientific findings, consider public comments, and develop the scientific report for updating the DGAs. The report is to be submitted to the Secretaries of HHS and USDA for HHS and USDA to consider as the Departments in developing the next edition of the *Dietary Guidelines*. The report is open for the public to view along with the new edition of the *Dietary Guidelines*.
4 **Step 4 – Develop the Dietary Guidelines.** The Advisory Committee submits its evidence review and recommendations to regulatory authorities responsible for the guidelines – the U.S. Department of Agriculture (USDA) and the Department of Health and Human Services (HHS). These departments may incorporate some, but not necessarily all, of the Advisory Committee's recommendations for the new editions. The decision to include recommendations is based on various considerations – e.g., policy priorities, economic factors, and practical challenges. Together, the HHS and USDA develop the new edition of the *Dietary Guidelines* that uses current evidence to build upon the preceding edition.
5 **Step 5 – Implement the Dietary Guidelines.** HHS and USDA release the updated *Guidelines* at the end of the 5-year updating cycle and work with Federal, state, and local partners to implement the new edition.

Details of this process across professional associations may vary, but the essential components in the process are widely shared – e.g., public involvement, expert scientific reviews, updating the guideline, communicating updates to practitioners or the public.

BOX 14.2 OUTSIDE PROFESSIONAL GUIDELINES

EBP requires health professionals to be critical consumers of practice guidelines. While guidelines cover common cases, they might not account for rare cases or cases that are complicated by co-morbidities or unusual circumstances. Moreover, evidence supporting a guideline might be weak or outdated. These realities may require the evidence-based practitioner to examine more recent primary studies or systematic reviews to inform decisions, advice, or actions.

Audiences for guidelines

As discussed, professional guidelines are based on the latest and best evidence available at the time they are written. They also may be written for different audiences to consume and use – i.e., health care professionals or the public at large.

Guidelines for the public are designed to provide accessible and easy-to-understand information for people to assimilate and use. They often focus on promoting healthy behaviors, preventing illness, and managing common health conditions. Examples include dietary guidelines, physical activity recommendations, vaccination schedules, and guidelines for managing minor illnesses or injuries at home. These guidelines are typically disseminated through public health campaigns, educational materials, websites, and community outreach programs. While written for the public, professionals often use them as tools to inform and educate clients regarding best practices.

Some guidelines are specifically written for health professionals to apply to treat or manage health conditions and are not available to the public. Guidelines for health professionals are typically more detailed and technical, accessible to the professional but not to the public at large. For instance, these include treatment protocols, algorithms for diagnostic testing, medication prescribing guidelines. These guidelines are often published in scholarly journals, in clinical practice guidelines databases, and professional society websites. We describe below guidelines published for physical therapists managing clients through total knee arthroplasty (see Examples 14.1 and 14.2).

Guidelines designed for use by health professionals

This type of guideline usually aims to provide detailed and specialized information to guide practice and ensure that health professionals have the most current and evidence to inform health decisions, advice, and actions. Written for professionals, they are described using terms that are familiar to the professional.

To illustrate, what follows describes a recommendation for guiding guide physical therapists in managing patients who have or will undergo a total knee arthroscopy (TKA).

Example 14.1   Management of patients who have undergone or will undergo Total Knee Replacement [1]

A guideline development team (from the American Physical Therapy Association) developed a guideline to inform physical therapists on how to manage patients who have or will undergo total knee arthroplasty (TKA). The guideline for prehabilitation or rehabilitation of TKA patients is based on systematic reviews along with other evidence.

The guideline highlights the burden of disease suggesting the importance of developing the guideline – e.g., the prevalence of chronic pain and disability due to knee osteoarthritis. The guideline offers evidence to guide different aspects of managing knee osteoarthritis. This includes, for instance, preoperative exercise and education, motor function training, post-operative knee range-of-motion exercises, resistance and intensity exercises, and prognosis.

While narrow in scope – actions the PT should take before and after TKA – the recommendation leaves considerable discretion to the professional to tailor decisions to suit the needs of the individual client. For instance, guidance for preoperative exercise broadly recommends that PT's should "design preoperative exercise programs and teach patients undergoing total knee arthroplasty (TKA) to implement strengthening and flexibility exercises" [1]. This is a broad charge, leaving the practitioner and client to discuss details surrounding training and exercise programs.

Guidelines identify how strong the evidence is that supports the recommendation so the professional may critically assess whether and how the guideline applies to a specific patient. For instance, evidence favoring the preoperative exercise recommendation to enhance strength and flexibility received 3 out of 4 stars and was rated as moderate. A moderate rating is defined as "…slight-to-moderate benefit, harm, or cost, or a moderate level of certainty for a moderate level of benefit, harm, or cost…". In contrast, the pre-op education program received just 1 star for – currently "best practice" – expert opinion and practice norms support the practice. The best practice appears safe and beneficial and seems better than known alternatives.

The professional is left to consider the strength of the evidence in shaping the recommendation in a way that suits the patients' health, living, and working situations (Box 14.3). For each recommendation, the guideline identified areas for future research and several years have passed since it was published. Where evidence supporting a recommendation is weak or moderate, the professional may consider searching for more recent primary studies or review studies to support their decisions.

BOX 14.3   STRENGTH OF RECOMMENDATIONS

A guideline for managing TKA attached degrees of obligation to follow the guideline based on the evidence supporting it [1]. For instance, a recommendation with high-quality evidence supporting it (e.g., systematic reviews, meta-analysis, and RCTs) "Must or Should" be followed (or avoided). In contrast, recommendations that are only supported by basic or bench science or expert opinion are less compulsory for the practitioner.

The next example is oriented toward public health teams, planning professionals, and local authorities, for promoting "healthy weight environments".

Example 14.2   Using the planning system to promote healthy weight environments: Guidance and supplementary planning document template for local authority public health and planning teams [2]

Public Health England put forward a plan for promoting equitable, healthy weight environments for local public health teams. This reflects an understanding that healthy weight environments can shape and foster more active lifestyles. The design principles are described in a larger narrative but depicted in the infographic shown in Figure 14.1.

The guidance aims to address a call from local public health teams for a planning system to foster an environment that supports a healthy weight for residents. A healthy

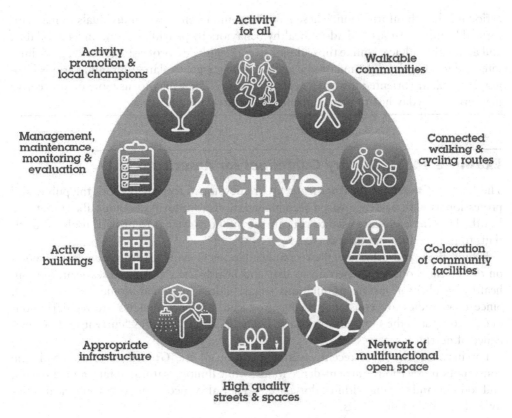

FIGURE 14.1   Ten design principles for promoting active lifestyles.

Source: Public Health England. Contains public sector information licensed under the Open Government Licence v3.0. https://assets.publishing.service.gov.uk/government/uploads/system/uploads/attachment_data/file/863821/ PHE_Planning_healthy_weight_environments_guidance__1_.pdf.

weight environment aims to advance health through prevention – e.g., by reducing obesity among adults and children.

The guidance is based on the research and experience of experts, presented within a national policy framework. While the recommendations are not based on evidence from RCTs or systematic reviews, the evidence supporting them was arguably the best available at the time.

Public health planners would incorporate these principles into their planning, often in collaboration with local authorities and tailored to local conditions. The evidence-based planner would tailor the recommendations to their client – the public and community. As always, other evidence from primary and review studies would be needed to update the evidence and address any gaps in the existing recommendation.

Guidelines designed for professionals and the public

Guidelines designed for use by both health professionals and the public are usually developed with the goal of promoting public health and wellness through accessible and actionable health information. These guidelines aim to empower individuals to make informed health decisions and adopt healthy behaviors by providing clear, understandable, and actionable advice. Unlike those designed for healthcare professionals only, guidelines intended for broader dissemination usually use language, explanations, and various infographics that are oriented toward a general audience. They may focus more on preventive measures, everyday health management, and lifestyle modifications.

Example 14.3 *Dietary Guidelines for Americans* [3]

The *Dietary Guidelines for Americans* [3] are developed to provide both the public and professionals with evidence-based recommendations to inform decisions about diet and health. The *Guidelines* are used to educate the public as well as to provide tools for dietitians to use in educating their clients.

Behind these and other dietary recommendations is evidence from numerous studies on the myriad topics that pertain to diet and health (e.g., chronic disease prevention, healthy weight) for various populations (e.g., children, pregnant women, older adults). Since new studies are constantly being produced, evidence reviews are regularly conducted to update the next edition of the *Guidelines* to reflect the "current body of evidence of nutrition sciences".

For instance, the most recent, available edition of the *Guidelines* recommends the consumption of various nutrient-dense foods, while limiting saturated fats, added sugars, and sodium, and staying within calorie needs. They also encourage regular physical activity and mindful eating habits.

Limiting added sugar intake to less than 10% of total daily calories was included as a recommendation in the 2015–2020 edition of the *Guidelines*. This version was based on an evidence review that linked the consumption of added sugar to several adverse health outcomes – e.g., obesity, type 2 diabetes, cardiovascular disease, and dental caries. The evidence reviews for the 2020–2025 *Guidelines* suggested that

> for adults and for children 2 years and older, a recommendation of less than 6% of energy from added sugars is more consistent with a dietary pattern that is both nutritionally and calorically appropriate, than is a pattern with less than 10% of energy from added sugars, as was recommended in past editions of the *Dietary Guidelines*.

Further refinements of the topic of the effects of added sugars will be addressed by the Dietary Guidelines Advisory Committee in an upcoming evidentiary review. The Committee will seek to answer the following question

> What is the relationship between food sources of added sugars consumed and growth, size, body composition, risk of overweight and obesity, and weight loss and maintenance, and risk of type 2 diabetes?

Thus, evidence reviews serve to both inform practice guidelines and identify gaps in our knowledge. These gaps help define the questions that future evidence reviews will seek answers to.

Recap

This chapter discussed professional practice guidelines – foundational tools in health care that offer evidence-based recommendations to guide practice decisions and actions. Developed by various regulatory agencies and professional associations, these guidelines capture a synthesis of the evidence based on a thorough and transparent review of current evidence. This synthesis flexibly guides practitioners and clients so decisions and actions can be tailored to accommodate the individual's preferences and circumstances.

The chapter also discussed cycles and processes for developing and updating practice guidelines – e.g., convening expert teams, reviewing current evidence, and making or revising recommendations. This ongoing process helps ensure that guidelines address pressing health concerns and incorporate new scientific evidence in a timely manner; where evidence is insufficient, the process serves to identify important areas where additional research is needed.

Finally, the Chapter provided examples to suggest how guidelines may be used in different contexts: managing patients undergoing total knee arthroscopy, planning a healthy weight environment, and adherence to the dietary guidelines for Americans. The examples illustrate how scientific research is used to inform evidence-based practice. They also show the limitations of our knowledge and, therefore, the importance of adapting what we do know to the unique particulars of the present situation.

References

1. Jette DU, Hunter SJ, Burkett L, Langham B, Logerstedt DS, Piuzzi NS, et al. Physical therapist management of total knee arthroplasty. *Phys Ther*. 2020; 100(9):1603–1631. 100. Available from: https://academic.oup.com/ptj.
2. Public Health England. Using the planning system to promote healthy weight environments: Guidance and supplementary planning document template for local authority public health and planning teams. 2020. Available from: https://assets.publishing.service.gov.uk/government/uploads/system/uploads/attachment_data/file/863821/PHE_Planning_healthy_weight_environments_guidance__1_.pdf.
3. U.S. Department of Agriculture and U.S. Department of Health and Human Services. *Dietary guidelines for Americans, 2020–2025*. 9th ed. 2020. Available from: DietaryGuidelines.gov.

PART 4

Topical Reading, Evidence-Based Practice (EBP), and Professional Growth

Part 4 discusses the fourth stage of reading – topical reading. Topical reading builds upon inspectional and analytical reading. Topical reading involves interpreting and synthesizing evidence from multiple studies on a specific topic to deepen understanding and inform evidence-based practice (EBP).

Chapter 15 offers a structured approach for organizing information extracted from the set of research studies that have been examined analytically. The chapter recommends the use of a literature review matrix to record key information extracted from these studies. The use of the literature review matrix fosters the comparison among studies, along with a unified interpretation of diverse findings. Consolidating evidence from multiple studies deepens one's understanding of the research evidence on a given topic.

Chapter 15 also emphasizes how topical reading is essential for EBP and patient-centered care. It fosters more informed discussion with patients and clients, encouraging the latter's engagement in the decisions and actions. The engagement of patients and clients is central to EBP. Further, the critical analysis and synthesis of health research not only enhances the professional's understanding of the health topic, but also contributes to professional growth and the continuous improvement of client outcomes. Over time, this cyclical process of reading and applying evidence encourages deeper engagement with EBP and highlights the significance of topical reading in health and healthcare.

DOI: 10.4324/9781003595663-18

15

TOPICAL READING, EBP, AND PROFESSIONAL GROWTH

Overview – topical reading

Topical reading is the fourth stage of reading. Topical reading occurs after several articles have been inspected and critically analyzed. Topical reading provides the professional with a broader and deeper understanding of the evidence about the topic. The process is shown in Figure 15.1.

During inspection, titles and abstracts that relate to the main research topic are inspected to determine which articles are relevant or not to the reader's aim. Articles deemed relevant are critically analyzed. As discussed in Parts 2 and 3, analytical reading involves asking questions about the methods, results, limitations, and implications of each study. Topical reading will then combine, compare, interpret, and, where possible, synthesize the evidence from these various studies.

Figure 15.1 also suggests the ongoing, cyclical nature of the reading process, suggesting the back and forth between inspection, analysis, and a broader comparative analysis and synthesis. Topical reading occurs throughout one's professional career – e.g., as professionals gain certifications and continuing education credits, when exploring a new or important health issue, or when migrating to another practice or specialty area.

Topical reading – interpreting and synthesizing two or more studies

Rarely is adequate understanding about a topic gained from the analysis of a single study. A second study can validate the findings of a first study if the evidence is consistent; if the evidence is inconsistent, it cautions against the application of the initial findings. Two or more studies can expand one's perspective on a topic, supplying evidence derived from different methods, populations, and settings. Multiple studies make a greater range of findings available to inform decisions. Topical reading involves the analysis and integration of evidence from two or more studies on a specific health topic.

For various reasons, topical reading may be required of health professionals. Emerging health threats (e.g., pandemics) about which clear practice guidelines or recent systematic

DOI: 10.4324/9781003595663-19

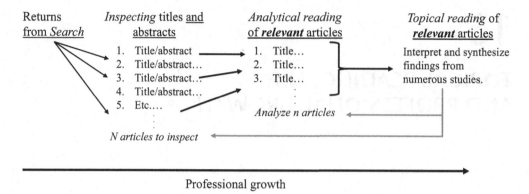

FIGURE 15.1   The reading process – inspection, analytic, and topical reading.

reviews are unavailable may require topical reading. Likewise, the development of innovative technologies may demand the analysis of several recent studies that offer evidence on how, where, and to whom they might apply or not. Clients and patients raise questions that the practitioner may not know the answer to that, therefore, may require the critical analysis of several studies. As discussed below, topical reading is central to professional growth and evidence-based practice.

Topical reading can often occur unsystematically without a clear plan or intent to collect and synthesize findings from various studies. Instead, research findings may be collected and analyzed in an ad hoc fashion, which is then interpreted and synthesized internally (in one's head). This passive approach is less effective, thorough, or precise than a more active approach would yield.

While few health practitioners will conduct their own systematic review, they still can be as systematic in how they explore a health issue or topic as time and energy will permit. A deliberate, systematic, and transparent approach will clarify what the evidence suggests about a health outcome, exposure, or health experience, thus helping to inform practice decisions. This is valuable even when current evidence is unclear or unreliable, as it acknowledges the limitations of our collective understanding of the topic and cautions us against the overzealous application of findings. This helps to promote honest communication, set realistic expectations, and cultivate shared decision making and personalized care.

A transparent, systematic approach to topical reading is aided by spreadsheet tools used to construct a matrix to guide the extraction and recording of information from various studies (Table 15.1). In this hypothetical topical reading matrix, each row represents an article to be read, and each column indicates the information one would extract from the article. The analytical questions described in earlier chapters may guide the process of populating the cells, but the columns used may be changed depending on the topic and what one wants to learn about it.

The takeaway

Use of the matrix elevates the transparency of the process and accumulates findings and takeaways as each study is added to the matrix. As articles are reviewed and rows are populated, one gains a deeper understanding of the methods used to study the topic – e.g., the designs,

TABLE 15.1 Sample topical reading matrix*

Citation (author, year)	—Article's Storyline—					Synthesis/ interpretation
	Objectives	Methods	Key findings	Limitations	Takeaway	
James et al. (2023)	To assess the association between dietary intact and blood pressure	Cohort Adults over 50; dietary intake; blood pressure adjusted HRs;	$n = 251$; χ age = 63.4; Med diet reduced risk of CVD, BP; aHR = 0.75	Excluded populations; unmeasured confounders;	Moderate support for an assoc. b/w veggie intake MED diet and lower CVD among older adults.	Synthesis of all articles; consistency of evidence; strength; credibility of theses
Johnson et al. (2021)	To test whether a dietary intervention reduces BP.	RCT 50 volunteers; 6-month diet intervention;	$n = 48$; ave. age = 41.4; BP reduced 12% in intervention group	Excluded populations; no blinding; artificial setting	MED diet intervention reduced BP among adults.	
.			.	.	.	
.						

* The citations and studies are hypothetical. The columns in this table are generic and will vary depending on topic and needs of the reader.

study populations, the measures, the analyses undertaken, and key findings. Each row serves to summarize a study. Taken together, the rows summarize all the studies.

Although studies differ in the research methods they use and the findings they produce, these differences are partially reconciled by describing findings and takeaways using similar terms. As much as possible, using similar terms fosters clearer comparisons of studies regarding the direction and strength of an association between health outcomes and exposures or the nature of experiences of health and illness. Results might all trend in the same direction, or they may differ and show gaps in our research and knowledge. Either way, the conclusion becomes clearer when takeaways are similarly described.

For instance, a cohort study may present an association between vegetable intake and cardiovascular disease (aHR = 0.75) whereas an RCT might show a 12% reduction in BP for a dietary intervention group. The results from the studies span 5 years and 6-months. These methods and results are somewhat different and must be harmonized with a common language. The common terms in each study pertain to health outcomes (CVD, BP) and exposure (dietary intake). Both studies examine this relationship among adults. The takeaways may be defined as

- "a cohort study over a 5-year period showed a moderate to strong association (aHR = 0.75) between vegetable intake and lower CVD among older adults" and
- "an RCT on the effects of a med diet intervention reduced BP by 12% among adults"

Adopting similar terms to characterize each takeaway – e.g., Med diet (exposure), CVD/BP (outcome), and adults (study populations) – will facilitate a consistent, unified interpretation and synthesis of the findings.

Interpretation and synthesis

Using shared terms in the takeaway for each study fosters a synthesis of the findings from the studies. In the example of dietary intake and cardiovascular disease, two different research designs are used: "observational and experimental studies provide evidence to support a relationship between diet and CVD/BP". Although aligning findings is more straightforward when the original studies use similar research designs, harmonizing evidence derived from different methods enhances our confidence in the reliability and credibility of the interpretation.

The topical reading matrix will likely include more than two studies, though it still may be limited to a handful of similar studies of high quality (Box 15.1). It is also the case that evidence from diverse studies may be inconsistent and more challenging to pull together, especially where different methods are used to generate the evidence. This challenges the professional to find common terms to enable a unified interpretation to be constructed. This result might suggest that the initial inquiry be refined or limited to a synthesis of fewer studies that use designs of a similar type.

Even when measures to refine the subject are taken, research results may be so incompatible that no unified interpretation develops. Learning what we do not know about a topic – the boundaries of our collective knowledge – is as valuable as learning what we do know. Understanding the limits of collective understanding facilitates honest communication based on evidence, shared decision making, personalized treatment, and patient or client autonomy.

BOX 15.1 FEWER STUDIES OF HIGH QUALITY

Topical reading does not require reading dozens of articles on the topic. During inspection, older and less relevant articles will be screened and excluded. During analytical reading, study methods will be further scrutinized for quality. Studies offering low-quality evidence can either be removed from the topical reading process, or their evidence can be de-emphasized when articles are compared and synthesized.

Topical reading and evidence-based practice (EBP)

This book mainly focuses on the critical analysis of health-related evidence, with topical reading as the highest form of evidentiary analysis and assessment. Topical reading and EBP are inextricably linked – topical reading involves the critical analysis of research evidence, and EBP involves the critical application of this evidence.

The application of evidence in the service of real, unique patient or client cases is often complicated. Each case is unique in terms of health history, personal circumstances, values, and priorities. A practice that is informed by current evidence must, therefore, account for how cases are similar to or different from the "average" case as suggested by research. Engaging with clients, therefore, is crucial for understanding their unique qualities and effectively applying the current evidence.

Patient and client engagement

EBP blends scientific understanding with the "art" of healthcare. Although discussion of the "art" of healthcare far exceeds our current scope, some general statements can be made regarding how client or patient engagement is crucial for EBP

1 **Initial assessment.** Standard assessment and screening tools provide a useful starting point for assessing the patient's status. Currency concerning the latest tools and what they offer is a central component of the initial assessment. Yet, patient engagement is required to collect information about the patient's condition and to assess the major health problem(s) the patient is experiencing and must manage. A more thorough conversation about the client's history – physical, mental, behavior, and social – provides a more complete picture of the patient's condition.
2 **Clarifying misconceptions.** Patient engagement requires an assessment of the patient's knowledge, values, and ability to manage or advance their own health. Patients hold misconceptions about their health that the EB practitioner will clarify. The professional's critical understanding of the latest health evidence is central to this task.
3 **Setting goals.**[1] Engagement enables the patient and practitioner to prioritize and co-define goals (desired health outcomes) for maintaining or advancing health. Goals may be viewed in short, medium, and longer terms. The EB practitioner will help the patient define these goals, making sure that they are realistic and that there are clear actions that the patient is able to take to achieve them.
4 **Developing a plan.** There are often different action options available for achieving the same goal. There are trade-offs associated with each option. Knee replacement surgery

carries inherent risks, but non-surgical options may require lifestyle changes, ongoing pain management, and the potential for surgery in the future. A goal to lose excess weight promises to reduce blood pressure and cardiovascular risks but may require changes in dietary habits that may contribute to fatigue, depression, or disordered eating. There is no easy way to attach value to the benefits and costs of these options. Only patients can properly weigh these options, as it is they who must carry out the plan and live with the consequences. The responsibility of the EB practitioner is to clarify these trade-offs so the patient can make an informed decision.

5 **Trust and Adherence.** Patient engagement elevates the patient's inclusion and trust throughout the healthcare process. Within a context of mutual trust, decisions about advancing the patient's health can be shared. While the individual patient may be the final decision maker, patients vary in their desire to fully participate in decisions, and many would rather defer to the practitioner's judgment (Box 15.2). Either way, actively engaging in the assessment, planning, and decision-making process enhances the patient's commitment to the resulting plan and the motivation and ability to follow it.

In short, while EBP involves the use of the best available evidence, patient engagement requires clear communication of this evidence to guide and inform patients. It also requires listening to patients to learn about their values, preferences, and health capabilities and collaborating to develop a plan to promote their health and well-being.

BOX 15.2   CLIENTS VARY

Ideally, it would be the fully informed client who, in collaboration with the professional, defines their health goals and plans to achieve them. Clients, however, vary in their tolerance for uncertainty and desire to make decisions. For instance, some are more health literate and are more confident than others in their ability to define and execute health plans. Some prefer to defer to the health professional presumed to possess expertise and to know what is best for them. Thus, an important task for the EB practitioner is to determine how active the client's wishes to be in the process of making decisions.

Reading, EBP, and professional growth

We discussed at the outset that critically reading health research is essential to evidence-based practice and professional growth. We introduced how to inspect article titles and abstracts to assess the relevance of an article to a particular aim. We described a process for analytically reading and assessing research articles (ten questions). Finally, we discussed topical reading where we might summarize or synthesize the findings and evidence pertaining to a health topic.

This chapter also touched on the importance of assessing how individual clients may resemble or differ from the general cases research evidence is based upon, along with the importance of exercising professional judgment when applying evidence to cases. Combined, the development of these skills underpins the process of professional growth. Figure 15.2 depicts how reading health research, EBP, and professional growth relate.

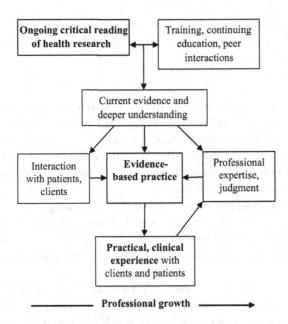

FIGURE 15.2   Reading, EBP, and professional growth.

The evidence base that informs EBP emerges from an ongoing critical reading and consumption of current evidence. While we narrowed our discussion to reading peer-reviewed research articles, professionals encounter evidence from various reports, online sources, professional conferences, and peer interactions. These other sources of evidence also deserve critical scrutiny.

Current evidence is, of course, fundamental to EBP. In view of the rapid output of primary and review studies, ongoing, critical reading of research is, correspondingly, fundamental. Command over current evidence is enhanced through ongoing training and education, and peer interactions in offices and conferences.

Yet this general evidence is typically applied one case at a time, with each case considered as unique. This poses a challenge to the EB practitioner, who then must adapt this general evidence to fit the specifics of each case. As discussed, the EB practitioner must interact with each case to build trust and gain understanding of their unique qualities. Some uncertainty surrounding decisions will remain, however, so health outcomes must be continuously monitored to allow adjustments to be made, and, importantly, to foster ongoing learning.

Practitioners learn from each new case – where and how evidence applies. This deepens their knowledge and understanding as they gain experience with each new, unique case. Over time, with experience, and with continuing education, the practitioner's judgment in applying general knowledge to unique cases becomes further refined. The cumulative effect is to nurture evidence-based practice, while it furthers professional growth.

Finally, from the process of critically reading health science, applying evidence, and learning from each new case, the cycle of EBP and professional's growth is reinforced. The cycle is initiated at the outset of and continues throughout one's professional career. As the habit of critically reading health research becomes cultivated, the beneficial effects for EBP and professional growth becomes increasingly evident in the quality of professional practice, and it materializes in the improved health of clients and patients.

Conclusion

In this exploration of the landscape of health research, we have outlined the process of elementary, inspectional, analytical, and topical reading to cultivate critical engagement with research evidence among students and health professionals. From primary studies to systematic reviews and practice guidelines, developing skills in critical reading and consuming research evidence is essential for health professionals committed to evidence-based practice for their clients.

Topical reading, the most advanced stage of critical reading, represents the practitioner's continuous effort to broaden and deepen their understanding of research evidence. It exemplifies a commitment to the health and well-being of their clients and underscores the importance of continuous learning in promoting health and healthcare of the highest quality.

Together, these chapters chart' a pathway for critically analyzing health research to inform evidence-based practice. They emphasize the crucial role of engaging critically with research evidence to encourage effective health practice while also supporting professional growth and development.

Reference

1. Franklin M, Lewis S, Willis K, Rogers A, Venville A, Smith L. Controlled, constrained, or flexible? How self-management goals are shaped by patient–provider interactions. *Qual Health Res.* 2018;28(4):573–584. doi:10.1177/1049732317753581.

APPENDIX A

Elementary reading and fundamental terms

Overview – basic terms of research methods

There is no getting around it – readers must learn and understand basic terminology required for reading health research. This is so self-evident that it can easily be overlooked. Learning basic terms of methods and topic-specific terms characterizes the first stage of reading. This stage of learning and expanding one's understanding of basic health research terminology continues throughout one's life and career. Over time, the professional's experiences will broaden, and the understanding of what terms mean will deepen.

As Chapter 1 describes, research articles contain terms that refer to a *topic* of interest (e.g., exposures, outcomes, or experiences) and those that refer to the principles and *methods* of research used to explore the topic. Topic-specific terms refer to the concepts associated with a substantive area of interest – e.g., wellness, public and population health, nutrition, kinesiology, and exercise science. Terms of research methods, however, are implicated in studying and expanding the evidence and knowledge on any health topic.

Elementary reading involves learning key terms one encounters during inspectional and analytical reading. Key terms are often understood through the contexts in which they are embedded and are readily looked up online. As a reference, however, several of these basic terms associated with research *methods* are described below.

Fundamental terms

- **"As if" randomization.** This is an assumption made in natural experiments where it is presumed that exposure to an event occurred "as if" at random, with no pre-existing differences present before it occurred. The assumption is then validated by other data to enhance its credibility. This also enhances the credibility of causal inferences made from the data.
- **Attrition.** This occurs when research participants do not complete the study – e.g., they are lost to follow-up, re-locate, or die. Participants who, for whatever reason,

drop out of the study may have different characteristics than participants who continue to the end. This represents a source of potential study bias (see Appendix B).

- **Confidence *interval* (CI)**. The confidence *interval* (CI) is the range of values, derived from the sample data, that is likely to contain the population parameter given a certain level of confidence. The interval reflects the degree of uncertainty around the estimate that researchers are willing to accept (see Appendix C).

- **Confidence *level***. The confidence *level* represents the degree of certainty (expressed as a percentage) that a series of confidence intervals constructed from multiple samples would include the true population parameter. Most studies are satisfied with a 95% level of confidence for estimating confidence intervals (see Appendix C).

- **Covariates**. Covariates are variables in a study that may affect the main exposure and outcome variables being studied. Covariates are statistically adjusted for to more accurately assess the relationship between exposures and outcomes.

- **Credibility (in qualitative research)**. Credibility has to do with how plausible the findings are, and how accurately they capture participants' experiences and perspectives. Credibility is gauged by the richness of the data and the quality of the analytical procedures used to limit biases.

- **Eligibility criteria**. Eligibility criteria define the qualities that sampling units (e.g., study participants, studies under review) must have or cannot have to be eligible for the study. These criteria are commonly referred to as the inclusion and exclusion criteria.

- **Ethics Review**. With ethics review, the research protocol and methods are fully described and submitted to an Institutional Review Board (IRB) for review before any data may be collected. Once the IRB approves the protocol, the study may proceed with data collection and analysis. IRBs are established in most research institutions to protect against unnecessary harm of research subjects. IRBs are referred to in different ways in different countries – e.g., Research Ethics Board (REBs), Research Ethics Committees (RECs), and Human Research Ethics Committees (HRECs).

- **Exposure**. The exposure is a variable seen to influence or "cause" change in a health outcome. For instance, observational studies might consider cardiorespiratory fitness, diet, physical activity, food security as exposures or risk factors associated with certain health outcomes. An experimental intervention is a specific type of exposure that the researcher introduces to affect health outcomes.

- **External validity**. External validity refers to the degree to which study results can be generalized to other populations, settings, or times. (Also see "internal validity".)

- **Hazard Ratios (HR)**. A statistic (ratio) used to assess the strength of an association between a health outcome and an exposure (see Appendix E).

- **Health Outcome**. A health outcome is any measure of health status or quality of life resulting from an exposure, risk factor, or treatment intervention. For instance, cancer rates, anxiety levels, weight loss, injury rates, test scores all vary across people and change over time. The health outcome can be seen as the "effect", "result", or "outcome" of changes in another variable.

- **Inductive analysis**. A primary mode of analysis for qualitative research where ideas and themes emerge organically from data collected rather than as pre-conceived ideas tested against the data.

- **Internal validity**. Internal validity refers to the extent to which the study methods effectively manage biases and allow for accurate causal inferences. (Also see "external validity").

- **Intervention.** Health interventions are a deliberate kind of exposure that researchers test, and health professionals use to affect health outcomes. Interventions are also referred to as experimental manipulations, treatments, programs, trials, and procedures.
- **Odds Ratios (OR).** A statistic used to assess the strength of an association between a health outcome and an exposure (see Appendix E).
- **Open Access.** Free, open access to academic literature to anyone with an internet connection.
- **P-value.** A statistic used to determine the likelihood that the observed relationship or difference in the sample occurred by chance (assuming the null hypothesis is true). The lower the p-value the lower the likelihood that the findings reported were due to random chance (see Appendix C).
- **Peer-reviewed articles.** Research articles that have been peer-reviewed are distinct subset of the vast universe of texts that make claims about health or illness. Peer-reviewed articles have been critically examined by experts in the field before being considered of sufficient quality to be published in a scholarly journal. To survive this critical scrutiny, peer-reviewed studies include a clear description of the methods used to enable readers to gauge the quality and limitations of the evidence presented. Evidence-based practice relies on evidence derived from peer-reviewed studies.
- **Pigeonholing.** The first action taken in inspectional reading. Pigeonholing an article refers to the act of classifying titles by their type into a limited number of categories – e.g., primary vs review study, quantitative vs qualitative approaches. It also involves parsing the title to identify the health outcome, population or group, or exposure being studied.
- **Point-estimate.** A statistic based on study observations that estimates the true value of the population parameter. For instance, the mean height of a sample of students would serve as a point-estimate of the average height in the student population.
- **Population parameter.** A population parameter is a number used to characterizes an entire population – e.g., 33% of the population is obese, life expectancy is 81 years, or 15% are atheists. Researchers use statistics to estimate the value of a population parameter based on the data from sample.
- **Precision.** The closeness repeated measures or estimates are to each other. This reflects the consistency of the set of values surrounding the sample statistic. The closer the measurements are to one another, the greater the precision.
- **Primary (original research) studies.** Primary studies are studies that either gather new data for analysis or assemble already-existing secondary data for analysis. Examples include studies that collect data from experiments, surveys, in-depth interviews, medical records, or databases that are publicly available. (see Chapters 5–11).
- **Qualitative studies.** Qualitative studies collect and analyze non-numeric data to capture experiences and perspectives on issues related to health, illness, and healthcare to improve our understanding of a particular population or phenomenon.
- **Quantitative studies.** Quantitative studies collect and analyze numeric data to understand the direction and strength of relationships (e.g., between health outcome and exposure). Quantitative studies use observational and experimental designs (see Chapters 5–9).
- **Response rate.** The response rate is based on the proportion of individuals selected to participate in a survey that responds. For instance, if 200 out of 1000 eligible participants completed a survey, the response rate would be 20%. A low response rate

may bias or limit the results, as respondents may differ from non-respondents in some significant way.

- **Review studies**. Review studies are studies of primary studies. They may also include other review studies or meta-analyses. Review studies describe, analyze, and synthesize results of the other studies. (see Chapters 12 and 13).

- **Risk Ratios (RR)**. A statistic (ratio) used to assess the strength of an association between a health outcome and an exposure. The risk ratio is also referred to as the "relative risk" (see Appendix E).

- **Sample statistic**. A study finding derived from data collection and analysis process and used to estimate a characteristic of the sample – e.g., 57% of the sample identify as women, the average age of the sample subjects is 21.3 years, the relative risk of injury of football players compared to baseball players is 2.32.

- **Standard deviation** (σ). The standard deviation is a measure of dispersion of data points around the mean value. It is computed as the square root of the variance (see Appendix C).

- **Trustworthiness (in qualitative research)**. Trustworthiness pertains to the transparency of the methods used to generate the findings, enabling the study to be replicated, confirmed, and the results transferred to other contexts. Results that are trustworthy are also credible.

- **Statistical adjustments**. Statistical adjustments are made to limit the effects of confounding covariates on outcomes and exposures. They are made to adjust for pre-existing differences in groups being compared. Adjusting for these imbalances helps clarify the relationship between the exposure and the outcome.

- **Variable**. A general scientific term to refer to anything that varies – any measured characteristic or attribute of people or things that varies or changes. Examples include age, annual income, blood pressure, any attitude or behavior, GPA, and test scores.

- **Variance**. A measure of dispersion of data points around the mean value. The variance is computed as the average of the squared differences between each point and the mean (see Appendix C).

- **Z-score or Standard score**. A measure that indicates how much a score for an individual case deviates from the mean score of all cases, expressed in terms of the standard deviation. The z-score may be positive or negative depending on whether the score for an individual case is above or below the mean.

APPENDIX B

Potential sources of bias

What follows are potential sources of biases often seen in research studies that can affect the validity of the results. It is important to highlight these as *potential* sources of bias, not necessarily *actual* biases within the specific study. Identifying actual biases would require a much more detailed analysis of a particular study. Nonetheless, awareness of potential biases adds uncertainty and reduces confidence in the study's results. Recognizing these biases enables health professionals to assess the limitations of study findings and how they might inform practice decisions.

This list of potential sources of study bias is not exhaustive but includes common biases that analytical readers should look for.

- **Attrition bias (dropout).** This occurs when research participants do not complete the study – e.g., they are lost to follow-up, re-locate, or die. Qualities of those who exit the study prematurely may differ substantially from those who remain. This also limits generalizability of the findings. Attrition is more problematic for studies that take place over an extended time.
- **Confirmation bias.** This is a type of researcher bias where the researcher's personal or disciplinary tendencies intentionally or unintentionally affect how they read and report the results of non-numeric text data. For instance, evidence that runs contrary to preconceived ideas might be downplayed or ignored, while evidence confirming these ideas are given extra weight in the interpretation. Qualitative studies and narrative reviews are particularly prone to this.
- **Confounding,** Confounding occurs when covariates interfere with and distort estimates of the association between the main health outcomes and exposures or interventions. The risk of confounding is particularly high when the sampling or assignment of subjects is not random.
- **Funding bias.** This is a particular type of bias that arises from conflicts of interests, where sources of funding affect the research process. Reliance on financial support, especially from private industry which have much to gain or lose from the research, can compromise various aspects of the study – its study design and implementation, the interpretation and reporting of results.

- **Hawthorne effect**. The Hawthorne effect involves change in health or behavior by participants due to their awareness of being observed rather than the intervention itself. For instance, a study comparing a new dietary program with standard dietary advice finds similar effects on weight loss, likely due to the Hawthorne effect. Having to report their dietary habits motivated participants in both groups to engage in healthy eating and physical activity.

- **Maturation**. Maturation has to do with change that naturally occurs for research subjects over time that may affect outcomes independently of the intervention. To manage this possible confounder, researchers will include a control group that is presumed to experience a similar maturation process. This helps isolate the effects of the intervention itself by enabling a meaningful comparison between groups.

- **Observer bias**. This occurs when the researcher's expectations affect their observations. This is most problematic for measures that require subjectivity. This can skew the data collection process toward favoring a particular result. *Blinding* researchers to group assignments can counter this bias.

- **Placebo effect**. Similarly, the placebo effect involves change in participants' health due to their expectations of the effects of the intervention rather than from the intervention itself. *Blinding* participants to their experimental group assignment can counter this bias.

- **Publication bias (in review studies)**. All review studies may suffer from "publication bias" – the tendency of journals to publish findings that support a relationship rather than findings that do not. While the risk of publication bias cannot be entirely avoided, tools are available to gauge the extent to which it might skew the results of the review. These tools are used in systematic reviews, but not in traditional, narrative review studies. Where present, publication bias will skew results toward identifying significant associations.

- **Pygmalion effect (aka the *Rosenthal* effect)**. This refers to the effects the researcher's expectations have on the behaviors of subjects. For instance, higher expectations from teachers often raise the performance of students.

- **Regression to the mean**. Regression to the mean is the tendency for unusually high or low values to migrate toward the average on subsequent measurements.

- **Researcher bias**. This occurs where researchers' unintentionally shape all aspects of the study process – data collection, analysis, and interpretation. Although researcher bias may occur in quantitative research, the risk is greatest in qualitative research. The heightened risk in qualitative research is mostly due to its reliance on subjective reports and interpretations as viewed through the eyes of both researchers and research participants.

- **Response bias**. This bias can arise from numerous sources. Response bias may result from poor recall, social desirability, misunderstood or poorly worded questions, question order, or interviewer bias (also see the Pygmalion effect and Self-report bias).

- **Rosenthal effect**. See the *Pygmalion* effect.

- **Selection bias**. This occurs when participants selected do not represent a broader population. This often results from non-random sampling or non-random assignment. For instance, health studies often rely on volunteers (self-selection) who arguably are particularly curious, motivated, or health conscious and, thereby, poorly represent the general population. It also occurs when certain participants drop out of a study (attrition bias). In review studies, selection bias occurs when inclusion/exclusion criteria inadvertently exclude relevant studies from the review and, thus, not all relevant evidence is taken into account ("cherry-picking").

- **Self-report bias**. This occurs when participants inaccurately report their own characteristics – e.g., attributes, behaviors, experiences, and outlooks. This bias may be due to mistaken memory (recall bias), misunderstood questions, or a desire to respond in a way that is more favorable than is the case (social desirability bias).
- **Test-retest bias**. Test-retest bias has to do with change in performance that can occur when the same test is repeated. This is mitigated by altering tests, or extending the time between tests.

APPENDIX C

Measures of central tendency and dispersion

There is nothing fancy or mysterious about descriptive statistics, but a number can say a lot (though far from everything) about what it represents. Descriptive statistics consist mainly of summary measures of central tendency – e.g., the mean, median, and mode – and measures of dispersion – e.g., frequencies, range, variance, and standard deviation. You are likely to be familiar with some of them, but a brief refresher is provided below.

Measures of central tendency

Measures of central tendency characterize the middle or average score in a study's sample. They often appear in a table in the Results section where demographic and other characteristics of the sample appear. For instance, often the first table tells the reader the average age of the participants, the frequency of the distribution of racial, ethnic, or gender attributes, education, and other baseline characteristics relevant to the study (e.g., BMI, co-morbidities, and behavioral attributes).

Measures of central tendency can capture, in a single statistic, the central value of a variable within a sample – i.e., the mean, median, or mode.

- **The mean**. The mean (average) value is the sum of the values for all cases in a sample, divided by the number of cases. For instance, the mean height of students in the classroom is 175 centimeters; the mean age is 21 years; the mean BMI is 25.3. The mean in some distributions might be dramatically affected by extreme values. For instance, the mean income of graduates from a certain high school class was $23 million mainly because one of its graduates became a billionaire. The mean value would be "skewed" upward. Since computing the mean requires dividing and summing values, the mean is only used for numeric variables.
- **The median**. The median value is the value of the "middle" case in a distribution, meaning that there are an equal number of cases that are lower and higher in the distribution. The median value is barely affected by either extremely high or low values. For

instance, the multi-billionaire in my graduating class dramatically skews the mean value but only marginally affects the median value, shifting the "middle" income slightly. The median and mean values are the same for perfectly "normal" distributions. The median is typically the preferred measure of central tendency for skewed distributions.
- **The mode.** The modal value is the most frequent or common value found in the distribution. If a sample includes 50 Christians, 20 Jews, 20 Muslims, 10 Hindus, 10 Buddhists, and 30 atheists, the modal religion would be Christianity.

Measures of dispersion

While the mean, median, and mode each provide a summary statistic to represent the center of the sample distribution, there also are statistics that summarize how values are dispersed across the distribution – e.g., how wide or narrow, spiked or flat, or skewed a distribution is. The most common measures of dispersion are the range, variance, and standard deviation.

- **The range.** The range is simply the difference between the highest and lowest values. For instance, if the height of the shortest student is 135 centimeters and the height of the tallest is 195 centimeters, the range would be 60 centimeters (195–135).
- **The variance.** Variance is a measure of how much values in a distribution differ from the mean value. The variance captures the spread or dispersion of values around the mean. The variance is computed by summing the squared differences between each data point and the mean, and dividing the sum by the number of values.
- **Standard deviation (σ).** Like the variance, the standard deviation is a summary measure of the dispersion of values around the mean. Statistically, the standard deviation equals the square root of the variance. Practically, the standard deviation is more frequently reported.

The commonly understood bell-shaped or "normal" distribution is used to help us understand the frequency and likelihood of cases deviating from the mean. The distribution is symmetrical, with the mean sitting at the center, and other values rest either higher or lower than the mean value. Values near the mean are more likely to occur, whereas values more distant from the mean are less frequent and probable. Outlying values sitting in the "tails" of the distribution are the least likely to occur.

Z-score (aka, standard score)

A z-score assesses how far a given case is from the average case, measured in terms of standard deviations. For instance, a tall person might have a z-score of 1.5, meaning the height is one and a half standard deviations above the mean. A short person might have a z-score of –1.0, meaning their height is one standard deviation below the mean. A person of average height would have a z-score of 0.0. A z-score for a particular value might be positive or negative, depending on whether the value is above or below the mean.

Z-scores are valuable for determining how much individual scores deviate from the mean value and are expressed in standard deviations. This standardization allows comparisons across variables measured in different units – e.g., height, weight, kilograms, inches, and centimeters. For instance, converting weights (in pounds) and heights (in inches) into z-scores enables a direct comparison between the two variables. Also, statistical procedures, such as correlational analysis, can then be used to assess the strength and direction (positive or negative) of the association irrespective of the units used to measure them.

Numeric and categorical variables

How variables are measured will affect the statistical operations used to analyze them. For instance, age may be assessed numerically as age in years (e.g., 0–100), and one can easily compute the mean age in a population. Similarly, age can be measured in terms of stages of life, such as infancy, childhood, adolescence, adulthood, or elderly. Measured in this way, it would not make sense to compute a mean age.

Often researchers consider four levels of measurement.

- **Binary or dichotomous variables**. Binary or dichotomous variables contain just two categories – e.g., yes-no, present-absent, case-control. For instance, injury status is classified as injured or not; experimental groups are classified as treatment or control; diabetes status is classified as either present or absent; toxic exposure is recorded as either exposed or not. Binary variables allow for no gradation or levels in the measurement of exposures or outcomes.
- **Nominal variables**. Nominal variables contain two or more distinct categories, but the categories are not ranked in any way. For instance, blood type is nominal variable that contains four categories – A, B, AB, and O. There is no ranking of blood types, say, as low, medium, or high. Other common unranked nominal variables include, religion, ethnicity, marital status, and gender identity (e.g., male, female, and non-binary). Nominal variables are, by their nature, unranked.
- **Ordinal variables**. Ordinal variables contain categories, but the categories are ranked, say, from low to high. For instance, blood pressure can be classified into categories such as low, normal, high-normal, and high blood pressure. Other common ordinal variables would be scales ranging from strongly disagree to strongly agree, educational attainment (HS, some college, college degree, and post-graduate), and risk levels (low, moderate, and high). Binary, nominal, and ordinal variables are sometimes also referred to as categorical variables.
- **Numeric variables**. Numeric variables such as height, weight, or blood glucose levels can be measured on a continuous scale. These variables are quantifiable and vary incrementally to allow for more precise measurement for analysis. Numeric variables are often referred to by other names – e.g., continuous, quantitative, interval, and ratio.

How variables are measured also affects the statistical operations used to assess a relationship between two variables. For instance, to assess the association between two nominal variables – e.g., gender and dietary preference – a chi-square statistic would be used. For a nominal and a numeric variable – e.g., gender and daily calorie intake – an analysis of variance (ANOVA) statistic would be used. For two numeric variables – e.g., daily calorie intake and weight – a Pearson correlation would be used.

Several statistical procedures test the relationship between variables, but you will find some to be more commonly seen in specific research areas.

APPENDIX D

Confidence intervals and statistical significance

Confidence intervals (CIs)

A sample statistic quantifies the value of a characteristic or property in the sample. By combining values of the sample statistic, the sample size, and the sample standard deviation, researchers can, with some level of confidence, estimate corresponding population parameters, such as the mean age or GPA in the target population. This estimate is expressed as a confidence interval (CI) with upper and lower limits surrounding the sample statistic – i.e., the range of values likely to include the population parameter.

The researcher can compute a CI that provides a range or interval within which the value of population parameter falls with some level of confidence. The formula for the 95% CI is

$$95\% \text{ CI} = \text{Sample statistic} \pm 1.96 * \left(\frac{\sigma}{\sqrt{n}} \right)$$

For instance, given the following information about the sample statistic, sample size, and standard deviation:

Mean weight $\bar{x} = 150$ pounds
Standard deviation $\sigma = 20$ pounds
Sample size $n = 100$ adults

The 95% CI is simply

$$95\% \text{ CI} = 150 \pm 1.96 * \left(\frac{20}{\sqrt{100}} \right) =$$
$$95\% \text{ CI} = 150 \pm 3.92$$

The upper limit of the 95% CI would be 153.92 pounds; the lower limit would be 146.08. While the best estimate of the average weight of adults in the population is 150 pounds, you can be 95% certain that the average weight falls somewhere between 146.08 and 153.92 pounds.

More generally, the CI is a function of the sample statistic and sample characteristics – the sample size and standard deviation. A larger sample (n) serves to narrow the CI and this means a more precise estimate. A larger standard deviation (σ) widens the CI and reduces precision. Intuitively this might make sense, but it is evident in the formula above.

Finally, the multiplier of ±1.96 – is based on the Z-score for a 95% confidence level (assuming that values are normally distributed and a sample size >30). Most analyses present results in terms of 95% CIs. To be 99% confident, the multiplier for the CI would be 2.58, thus expanding the CI. The use of 99% CIs is more likely in areas of research where the consequences of being incorrect are severe.

BOX D.1 SAMPLING ERROR (SE) AND STANDARD ERROR OF THE MEAN (SEM)

Sampling error arises from inherent variation ("error") in the sample selection process. Sampling error refers to the difference between the sample statistic and the population parameter. Since the exact population parameter is often unknown, sampling error cannot be directly measured. However, the standard error of the mean (SEM) can be calculated to quantify how precisely the mean estimates the population mean. The SEM is like the CI in using the sample standard deviation (σ) divided by the square root of the sample size (n) to estimate the precision and reliability of the sample statistic – $SEM = \dfrac{\sigma}{\sqrt{n}}$.

Understanding statistical significance and "p-values"

The null hypothesis (H_0) asserts that there is no association between two variables – the two vary randomly, with no meaningful connection. In contrast, a second, alternative, hypothesis (H_a) asserts that a meaningful relationship might exist between the variables – variation in one variable is associated with variation in another. Which hypothesis does the data support?

To answer this, researchers test the probability that the observed association between the variables occurred by chance. This probability is expressed as a "p-value", which can range from 0.00 (impossible) to 1.00 (absolute certainty). Since anything is possible and nothing is certain, that p-value falls somewhere in between.

- If the data suggests that the observed association was probably due to chance, then the null hypothesis (H_0) is supported, and the alternative hypothesis (H_a) is not.
- If the data indicate a low probability that the association occurred by chance ($p \leq 0.05$), then H_0 is rejected, and H_a receives support.

A threshold or "alpha" level is set to identify when the null hypothesis should be rejected in favor of the alternative research hypothesis. Commonly, studies set this threshold or p-value to $p \leq 0.05$ (see Box D.2). An association where $p \leq 0.05$ would be considered "statistically significant" – i.e., there is less than a 5% likelihood that the observed association occurred by chance. If the p-value of an observed association is $p \leq 0.05$, this would indicate that it was unlikely (less than 5% chance) to have occurred by chance. The null hypothesis would be rejected in favor of the alternative hypothesis.

BOX D.2   WHY $p = .05$?

The use of $p = 0.05$ as the alpha level is mainly based on historical precedent and current convention. It has become a standard for publication. It also strikes a desired balance between the risk of committing a Type I error – falsely rejecting the null in favor of the alternative hypothesis – versus committing a Type II error – falsely retaining the null hypothesis and, thus, missing a true association. For instance, if missing a true positive is costly (e.g., when a miss has dire consequences), the threshold might be lowered. Similarly, if the cost of too many false negatives is high, lowering the threshold – e.g., to $p = 0.01$ – may be advised.

APPENDIX E

Tests of statistical significance – Chi-Squares, *t*-tests, and ANOVAs

Three tests commonly used to assess whether differences are likely due to chance are the chi-square test, the *t*-test, and the analysis of variance (ANOVA). The chi-square test is used to compare two categoric variables. The *t*-test is used to compare two groups along a continuous variable. The ANOVA is a more generalized version of the *t*-test, allowing comparison between more than two groups along a continuous variable.

Chi-square (χ^2)

The chi-square test is used to test whether the observed difference between two categorical variables is likely to have occurred by chance. Categoric variables may consist of two or more of categories – e.g., gender, ethnicity, blood pressure (low, normal, high).

For instance, the chi-square statistic could be used to test whether smokers who participated in the smoking cessation program were as likely to quit smoking as those who did not. The null hypothesis (H_o) is that both groups are equally likely to quit smoking. The research hypothesis (H_a) is that the groups are not equally likely to quit but, rather, that the cessation program will work (H_a). The *p*-value measures the likelihood that observed differences were due to chance. If the *p*-value is low, then we can rule out chance as a plausible explanation for the differences. In this example, $p < 0.01$, suggesting that the differences are statistically significant, and the data support H_a (Table E.1).

The chi-square test may be used with categorical variables that include more than two categories as well. For instance, the chi-square test can determine whether food security status (very low, low, marginal, high) is evenly distributed across socioeconomic status groups (low, medium, high) or whether observed differences were large and unlikely due to chance (e.g., $p < 0.05$) enough to be deemed statistically significant.

TABLE E.1 Effect of program participation on smoking cessation

Program participation	Quit smoking	Did not quit	Total
Participated	80	20	100
Did not participate	40	60	100
Total	120	80	200

$p < 0.01$

t-test

The t-test (aka the "Student" t-test) assesses how likely it is that an observed difference between two means (mean differences) was due to chance. Using a t-test to compare means requires that: (a) one of the variables is continuous so a mean can be computed, and (b) two (and only two) means are being compared.

A t-test might compare two means from two different samples. For instance, a t-test can compare whether the mean test performance between women and men is the same or significantly different (e.g., $p < 0.05$). This comparison is referred to as an "independent samples" (or "unpaired) t-test.

A t-test might also compare two means that come from the same subjects observed at two times – e.g., before and after an intervention. This before-after comparison is referred to as a "paired sample" t-test. For instance, a t-test might determine whether differences in knowledge scores before and after a dietary management program were due to chance or were significantly different (e.g., $p < 0.05$).

Analysis of Variance – ANOVA

ANOVA is a generalized form of a t-test. While a t-test is used to compare means of two groups, ANOVA (Analysis Of Variance) is used to compare three or more groups. For instance, if the observed change in anxiety scores is the same across intervention groups A, B, and C, ANOVA would show no significant difference in the average scores among the groups. However, if the change in anxiety scores for those exposed to intervention A was significantly different ($p < 0.05$) from groups B and C, this suggests that the difference is unlikely due to chance. Instead, it supports the conclusion that intervention A was effective in reducing anxiety.

APPENDIX F

Strength of association

A relationship might be statistically significant but weak and of little importance for practice decisions. For instance, a study might find that one diet reliably contributes to a 3-pound weight loss over 12 months, while another diet contributes to a 10-pound weight loss in 6 months. Both results may be statistically significant, but the second diet shows a stronger effect and is of greater practical significance. That is why it is important to also consider how strong the relationship is between the exposure and outcome or the size of the effect of an intervention on an outcome.

Chapter 5 describes how Pearson r correlation is used to capture an association between two continuous or numeric variables. The value of Pearson r ranges from -1.0 to 1.0; a Pearson r of 0.0 indicates zero association between two variables. The Pearson r statistic is often interpreted as showing a weak, moderate, or strong relationship. As a rule, Pearson r ranging from 0.00 to ± 0.30 is considered to be a modest or small correlation; a Pearson r between $= \pm 0.30$ to ± 0.70 is considered as a "moderate" correlation; a Pearson $r \geq \pm 0.70$ is interpreted as a strong correlation between the variables.

While Pearson r captures the relationship between two continuous variables, odds ratios (ORs), risk ratios (RRs), and hazard ratios (HRs) capture the strength of association between two binary or dichotomous variables. Cohen's d and the standardized mean difference (SMD) are used to assess the strength of the relationship between a binary variable (e.g., an experimental or control group) and a numeric variable to capture the size of a difference or an effect. What follows is a brief overview of these measures of effect size.

Ratios

Ratios are statistical measures used to assess the relationship between health outcomes and exposures that are measured as binary variables – e.g., present or absent, yes or no, dead or alive. These ratios compare two groups that differ in terms of health outcomes or health exposures. Specifically, odds ratios (ORs) are used in case-control studies where groups with or without an outcome present are compared with respect to exposures. Risk ratios (RRs) and Hazard ratios (HRs) are often used in cohort studies that compare

TABLE F.1 Odds ratio – Liver disease and reported alcohol
consumption

		Liver disease		
		YES	NO	
Reported alcohol	High	225	75	300
consumption	Low	75	225	300
		300	300	600

groups based on level of exposure in terms of health outcomes that may subsequently arise. These measures are often "adjusted", statistically, to account for potential confounders and to enhance the accuracy of the results.

Odds ratios

An OR is a ratio of two odds – the odds of those with an outcome (e.g., a disease or condition) having a been exposed, divided by the odds of those without an outcome having been exposed. For instance, a research team decided to match 300 people with liver disease (cases) with 300 people without liver disease (controls) to compare alcohol exposure in the two groups. Alcohol exposure was divided into two categories – high alcohol consumption and low/no alcohol consumption. Alcohol consumption is measured as a binary variable, rather than an ordinal or numeric variable. This study yielded these hypothetical results:

The OR is a ratio of ratios. Starting with the 300 respondents (cases) with liver disease – what are the odds they reported being heavy alcohol consumers? The calculation is straightforward:

$$\text{Odds } \textbf{\textit{with}} \text{ liver disease} = \frac{225}{75} = 3.0 \tag{1}$$

In other words (equation #1), subjects with liver disease are three times more likely to report high alcohol consumption than low alcohol consumption.

What are the odds that respondents without liver disease report being heavy alcohol consumers? The frequencies are different, but the calculations are similar to those in equation #1:

$$\text{Odds } \textbf{\textit{without}} \text{ liver disease} = \frac{75}{225} = .33 \tag{2}$$

In other words (equation #2), respondents without liver disease (controls) are one-third as likely to report heavy alcohol consumption compared to low alcohol consumption.

Next, the OR is simply the ratio of these two odds:

$$\text{Odds } \textbf{\textit{ratio}}, \text{ or OR} = \frac{3.0}{.33} = 9.0 \tag{3}$$

In other words, for Equation #3, the OR is a whopping 9.0 – people with liver disease are nine times more likely to report high alcohol consumption than people without liver disease.

When the number in the numerator (odds of exposure among cases) is greater than the number in the denominator (odds of exposure among controls), then the OR must be greater than 1.0. In the example, the odds of reporting high alcohol consumption are 9.0 times greater for subjects with liver disease compared to those without liver disease. Other times the OR might be lower than 1.0. For instance, if people with heart disease (cases) are less likely to follow a vegetarian diet than controls without heart disease.

Finally, when the numerator and the denominator are the same – i.e., when cases and controls have an equal likelihood of being exposed – the OR would equal 1.0. An OR of 1.0 indicates no association between the outcome and the exposure. To assess the strength of an association, you can check how far the OR deviates from 1.0.

Risk Ratios (RRs) and Hazard Ratios (HRs)

Both ORs and RRs both compare one group to another, though the groups being compared are slightly different. As discussed, ORs compare cases where the outcome is present to controls where the outcome is absent in terms of prior exposures or risk factors. ORs are commonly used in case-control studies. In contrast, RRs (also called relative risks) compare exposed and unexposed groups (cohorts) in terms of subsequent health outcomes. RRs reflect observations made forward in time to capture the risks and benefits of various exposures, interventions, and behaviors on health outcomes. For instance, a study might track soccer and basketball players during a season to determine if the risk of injury is higher in one sport compared to another. Examples 7.3 and 7.4 also illustrate the cohort design.

The hazards ratio (HR) is a close cousin to the RR and often is understood in a similar way, comparing the risk of some health outcome (e.g., sickness, injury, death) between exposed and unexposed groups. Unlike RRs, however, HRs assess not only if an outcome occurred but also when it occurred within the study period. For instance, in a cohort study that compared mortality outcomes for smokers and non-smokers, HRs account for whether mortality for smokers or non-smokers occurred earlier or later.

Summary of ratios

ORs, RRs, and HRs share similar characteristics:

1 They are all based on two binary variables measured in terms of the presence or absence of an exposure or an outcome;
2 These measures are calculated as a ratio of ratios. For instance, an RR captures the likelihood of an event occurring in the exposed group compared to the unexposed group.
3 Ratios equal to 1.0 indicate that there is no difference between exposed and unexposed groups in terms of outcomes (for RRs and HRs) or between cases with or without the outcome in terms of exposures (for ORs);

4 The farther the ratio is from 1.0, the greater the difference between the two groups, and the stronger the association between variables.

There are some differences between OR, RR, and HR statistics

5 ORs are mainly used in case-control studies to compare the odds of an exposure between cases with the outcome and controls without the outcome. In contrast, RRs and HRs are used in cohort or experimental studies to compare the risk of an outcome occurring between exposed and unexposed groups.
6 RRs and HRs are both concerned with comparing the risk of outcomes between exposure groups. RRs compare the overall risk of an outcome occurring between exposure groups without considering the timing of the event. HRs add a temporal dimension to the assessment of risk. This is especially relevant in studies where the 'when' is just as important as the 'if', allowing HRs to provide a dynamic measure of risk over time.

Standardized mean differences (SMD) – Cohen's *d*

A standardized mean difference or SMD is used to compare how two groups change along a continuous variable. The SMD quantifies the difference in means between the groups in term of standard deviation units. This makes the SMD useful for comparing the effect sizes of interventions across different studies. Cohen's *d* is one in a handful of SMD statistics (e.g., Hedge's *g*, Glass's Δ) commonly used to measure average group differences or change in outcomes between groups.

For instance, a researcher might wish to assess the effectiveness of an intervention designed to reduce anxiety, measured on a scale from 0 to 20. If the mean anxiety score decreased from 12 to 8 in the treatment group and stayed the same in the control group, then the average effect on anxiety would be 4 points. However, if anxiety scores fluctuate considerably, a 4-point difference would be less meaningful than if anxiety scores were more stable and clustered around the mean.

Cohen's *d* takes the dispersion of scores into account by pooling the standard deviations of the groups

$$d = \frac{\bar{x}_1 - \bar{x}_2}{SD_{pooled}}$$

where $\bar{x}_1$ is the mean score of the first group, $\bar{x}_2$ is the mean score of the second group, and the SD_{pooled} is the combined standard deviation of the two groups.

The value of Cohen's *d* must be interpreted. A Cohen's *d* of zero (0) indicates that there is no difference in means between groups – zero effect size. A larger Cohen's *d* suggests a larger effect size. But how large is large? Table E.2 shows conventional guidelines.

These guidelines are based on convention and should be interpreted within the specific context of the research, the nature of the intervention and outcome being examined, and the practice decisions to which the findings might apply.

TABLE F.2 Guidelines for gauging the size of an effect as indicated by Cohen's *d* scores

Cohen's d score*	Understood as
0.00–0.20	**Small effect** – the intervention appears to affect the outcome, but the effect may not be meaningful
0.20–0.50	**Moderate effect** – the intervention appears to affect the outcome, possibly enough to consider when making a decision
0.50–0.80	**Large effect** – the intervention appears to have a large effect on the outcome, and should be considered consider when making a decision
0.80–1.20	**Very large effect** – the intervention appears to have a large effect on the outcome, and should be considered consider when making a decision
>1.20	**Exceedingly large effect** – the intervention appears to have a large effect on the outcome and should be considered consider when making a decision

* These ranges apply irrespective of the direction of the effect (i.e., either positive or negative).

Summary of Cohen's d

1 Cohen's *d* measures the standardized mean difference in outcomes between groups, expressing the size of the intervention's effect;
2 a Cohen's *d* of zero (0) indicates that the intervention has no effect on the outcome, whereas values further from zero (in either direction) have increasingly meaningful effects.

INDEX

Note: **Bold** page numbers refer to tables and *italic* page numbers refer to figures.

Printed in the United States
by Baker & Taylor Publisher Services

Printed in the United States
by Baker & Taylor Publisher Services